Permar's

Oral Embryology and Microscopic Anatomy

A Textbook for Students in Dental Hygiene

TENTH EDITION

Frontispiece. Photomicrograph of a ground section cut faciolingually through a human maxillary first premolar (very low power magnification). The enamel contains a deep fissure in the central developmental groove. At the entrance to the fissure, on the triangular ridge of the buccal cusp, a barely visible dark area can be seen. This is most likely the beginning of a caries lesion, but there is no evidence of caries at the bottom of the fissure.

In the enamel on the buccal and on the lingual surfaces of the crown, the narrow light and dark areas of the bands of Hunter-Schreger may be faintly seen near the dentinoenamel junction.

Notice the curvature of the dentinal tubules in the crown of the tooth and the configuration of the pulp chamber: the pulp horn in the buccal cusp extends much farther occlusally than the pulp horn in the lingual cusp. In this photo, the pulp cavity is empty because the pulp tissue was destroyed during tissue preparation. Notice the relatively narrow root canals. It is difficult to determine the thickness of the cementum on this section at this magnification.

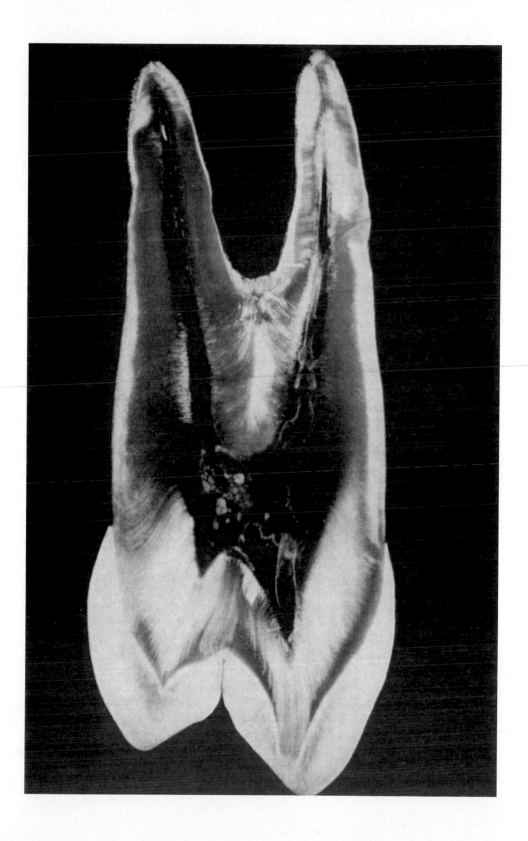

Permar's

Oral Embryology and Microscopic Anatomy

A Textbook for Students in Dental Hygiene

TENTH EDITION

Rudy C. Melfi, DDS, PhD

Professor Emeritus
Department of Oral Biology
College of Dentistry
The Ohio State University
Columbus, Ohio

Keith E. Alley, DDS, PhD

Professor
Department of Oral Biology
College of Dentistry
The Ohio State University
Columbus, Ohio

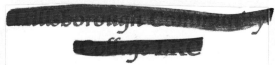

 LIPPINCOTT WILLIAMS & WILKINS

A **Wolters Kluwer** Company

Philadelphia • Baltimore • New York • London
Buenos Aires • Hong Kong • Sydney • Tokyo

Editor: Larry McGrew
Managing Editor: Angela Heubeck
Marketing Manager: Debby Hartman
Production Editor: Lisa JC Franko

351 West Camden Street
Baltimore, Maryland 21201–2436 USA
530 Walnut Street
Philadelphia, Pennsylvania 19106–3621 USA

Printed in china

First Edition, 1955
Second Edition, 1959
Third Edition, 1963—Reprinted, 1965
Fourth Edition, 1967—Reprinted, 1969
Fifth Edition,1972—Reprinted, 1973, 1975
Sixth Edition, 1977—Reprinted, 1979, 1980
Seventh Edition, 1982—Reprinted, 1985
Eighth Edition, 1988
Ninth Edition, 1994—Reprinted, 1995, 1996

Library of Congress Cataloging-in-Publication Data

Melfi, Rudy C.
    Permar's oral embryology and microscopic anatomy: a textbook for students in dental hygiene.—10th ed. / Rudy C. Melfi, Keith E. Alley.
        p.; cm.
    Includes bibliographical references and index.
    ISBN 978-0-683-30644-6
    ISBN 0-683-30644-8
    1. Teeth—Histology.   2. Mouth—Histology.   3. Embryology, Human.   4. Dental assistants.
I. Title: Oral embryology and microscopic anatomy.   II. Alley, Keith E.   III. Permar,
Dorothy. Permar's oral embryology and microscopic anatomy.   IV. Title.
    [DNLM: 1. Mouth—embryology.   2. Tooth—anatomy & histology. WU 101 M521p 2000]
RK280 .P4 2000
611′.018931- -dc21

                                                                                    00-021829

The publishers have made every effort to trace the copyright holders for borrowed material. If they have inadvertently overlooked any, they will be pleased to make the necessary arrangements at the first opportunity.
    To purchase additional copies of this book, call our customer service department at **(800) 638-3030** or fax orders to **(301) 824-7390.** For other book services, including chapter reprints and large quantity sales, ask for the Special Sales department.
    For all other calls originating outside of the United States, please call **(301) 714-2324**.
***Visit Lippincott Williams & Wilkins on the Internet:* http://www.lww.com**. Lippincott Williams & Wilkins customer service representatives are available from 8:30 am to 6:00 pm, EST, Monday through Friday, for telephone access.

7 8 9 10 11

RRS0912

For

DOROTHY PERMAR

Late Professor of Dentistry
The Ohio State University

Preface

This edition of *Permar's Oral Embryology and Microscopic Anatomy* is enhanced by the co-authorship of Keith E. Alley. His knowledge of and participation in dental education and research brings fresh insight and expertise to the book.

This book was written for students who have selected Dental Hygiene and Dental Assisting as career goals. Because these students have so much to learn, in so many subjects, presenting them with detailed accounts of complicated physiologic processes would not serve to broaden their education. Instead, it would place them in a maze. With this in mind, the text has been kept simple enough to be understandable and comprehensive enough to be useful.

It is assumed that the student who uses this book has taken a course in biology and has some knowledge of both mammalian anatomy and human tooth morphology. Although it would be helpful, comprehensive instruction in histology or embryology is not necessary.

The subject matter includes an introduction to general histology; the embryologic development of the face and oral cavity; development of teeth and their eruption and, in the case of primary teeth, their shedding; tooth enamel, dentin, cementum, and pulp; periodontal ligament; oral mucosa; gingiva; salivary glands; developmental tooth anomalies; dental caries; and a chapter on the temporomandibular joint.

A vital part of this book is the photomicrographs and illustrations. They help in the interpretation of the written content, which at times may be difficult to follow without visual aids. For further amplification of the material, new color photographs with succinct figure descriptions have been added to the tenth edition. It is anticipated that they will arouse the visual senses and provide vivid views of the tissues.

Students interested in exploring the literature for information in greater depth will find the references at the end of chapters to be helpful. References have been selected from publications usually available to students of dentistry and dental health. The references are by no means exhaustive, and those cited should be considered guideposts for the beginning student who seeks additional information on a particular subject.

We are grateful for the courtesies of our associates. Their names appear in association with figures throughout the book.

Rudy C. Melfi and Keith E. Alley
Columbus, Ohio

Contents

Color Plates

The color plates contained herein
are reproduced in black and white
in their corresponding chapters.

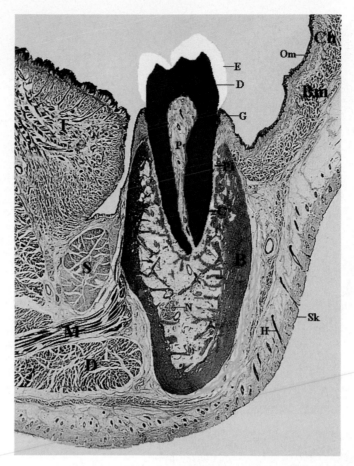

Figure 1–1. Photomicrograph of a frontal section through the mandibular second premolar. This picture shows the interdependent relationships among the tissues that make up the components of the oral cavity. Structures derived from epithelial tissue: OM, oral mucosa; G, gingiva; SK, skin; H, hair follicle; S, salivary gland; E, enamel of the tooth. Connective tissue derivatives: B, bone of the mandible; PL, periodontal ligament; CH, connective tissue of the cheek; D, dentin of the tooth; C, cementum of the tooth; P, dental pulp. Muscle tissue derivatives: T, tongue muscles; D, digastric; M, mylohyoid; Bm, buccinator. Nerve tissue derivative: N, inferior alveolar nerve that innervates the teeth, lips, and gums.

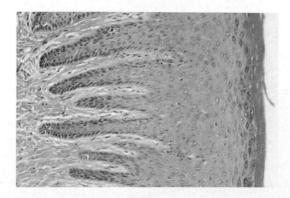

Figure 1–5. Photomicrograph of an oral mucous membrane section. A darker-stained stratified squamous epithelium is interdigitating with and connected to an underlying lighter-stained fibrous connective tissue. The surface layer of the epithelium is keratin. Compare to Figs. 1-2 (p. 5) and 1-6 (p. 11).

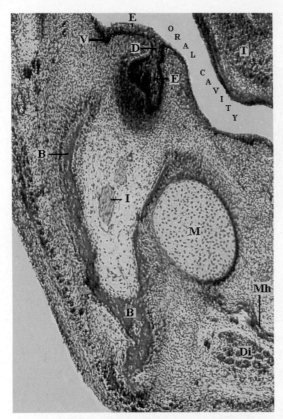

Figure 3–5. Frontal section of one side of a lower jaw in the region of the developing primary first molar, 8-week human embryo. Note the densely packed mesenchymal cells adjacent to the early epithelial enamel organ (cap); these cells will become the dental papilla and dental sac of the tooth germ. T, tongue; E, oral epithelium; V, vestibular lamina; D, dental lamina; E, early enamel organ or cap stage of tooth development; B, bone of developing mandible; I, inferior alveolar nerve; M, Meckel's cartilage; MH, mylohyoid muscle; DI, digastric muscle.

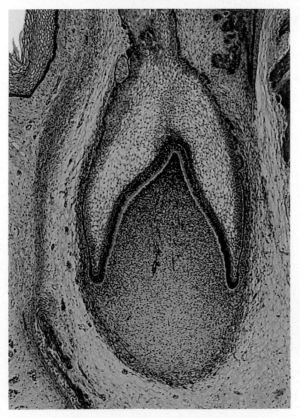

Figure 3–7. Photomicrograph of a faciolingual section of a lower incisor tooth germ. The bell-shaped enamel organ encloses the densely arranged mesenchymal cells of dental papilla. A lightly stained basement membrane lies between the enamel organ and the dental papilla and marks the future site of the dentinoenamel junction.

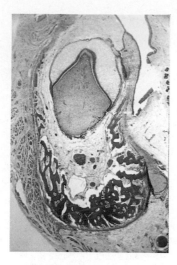

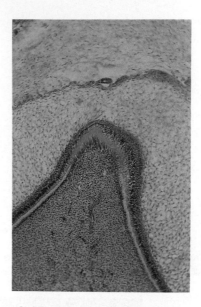

Figure 3–16. Microscopic view of the human mandibular incisor tooth germ. This tooth germ is more advanced in development than the tooth germ seen in Fig. 3-14 (p. 55). Dentin, the first mineralized tissue to appear in the tooth germ, is present at the coronal most part of the densely cellular dental papilla. The four cell layers of the enamel organ enclose the dentin and the cells of the dental papilla. From the lower edge of the photo to the apical part of the tooth germ is the spongy bone pattern of the mandible. The prominent round structure seen apical to the tooth germ and within the developing mandible is the inferior alveolar nerve. A higher magnification of the coronal part of the tooth germ is seen in Fig. 3-17 (at right).

Figure 3–17. Higher magnification of the coronal part of the developing tooth seen in Fig. 3-16. The first layer of dentin is clearly seen within the topmost part of the dental papilla. The four epithelial cell layers of the enamel organ surround the dentin and the densely packed cells of the dental papilla. Refer to Fig. 3-18 (p. 59) for orientation and identification of tissues.

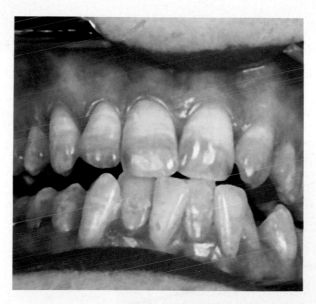

Figure 3–35. Clinical view of mottled enamel or dental fluorosis. Note that the teeth appear normal except for the brown-stained, hypomineralized areas caused by excessive exposure to fluoride during the period of enamel formation.

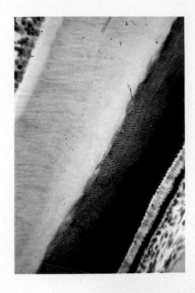

Figure 4–13. A demineralized section of an area of forming enamel and dentin. The dark-stained acid-resistant enamel lies adjacent to the lighter-stained dentin. Ameloblasts are seen along the enamel surface (lower right), and odontoblasts are along the pulpal surface of dentin (upper left).

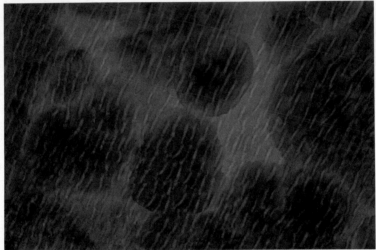

Figure 5–14. Microscopic view of a demineralized section of crown dentin, cut through areas of interglobular dentin. The dark-stained globular areas are mineralized; the lighter-stained, irregularly shaped areas of interglobular dentin are unmineralized. Note that parts of dentinal tubules are found throughout globular and interglobular areas. Compare to the ground section in Fig. 5-13 (p. 125).

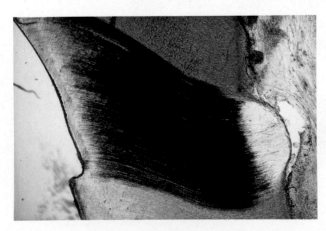

Figure 5–18. Microscopic view of an area of dentin beneath a surface (left) that was cut to receive a filling. Clearly visible is a dead tract, where the dentinal tubules are void of cell processes and are darkened because of the presence of air. Pulpal to the dead tract is a clear area of reparative dentin protruding into the pulp cavity on the right.

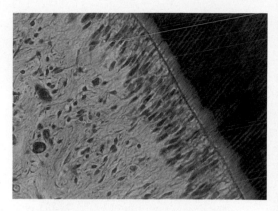

Figure 6–4. Higher magnification of an area of pulp and dentin. The prominent cell bodies of the odontoblasts are arranged along the lighter-stained predentin layer. On close inspection, the odontoblast cell processes are seen passing into the dentinal tubules.

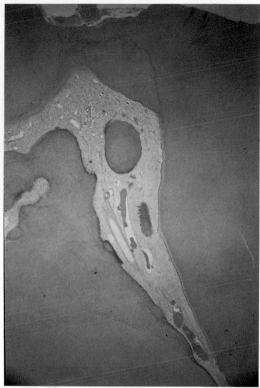

Figure 6–11. Longitudinal section of an old human molar. The tissue of the pulp chamber (above) continues into a root canal (below). A large pulp stone (denticle) in the pulp chamber is surrounded by pulp tissue that contains age-related changes (e.g., fewer cells, a deeply stained intercellular substance indicating an alteration of the organic components, possibly an increase of collagen fibrils, and pulpal mineralization). Notice the prominent blood vessels, some of which are engorged with blood cells.

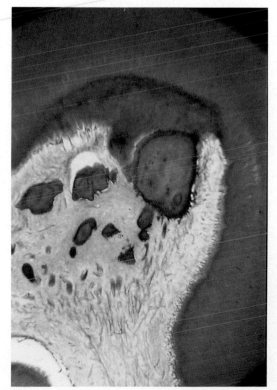

Figure 6–13. Photomicrograph of a section through the pulp chamber of an old molar tooth. Pulp stones of different sizes and shapes are visible. A large pulp stone is attached to the pulpal wall of the dentin. Notice the age-related changes in the pulp.

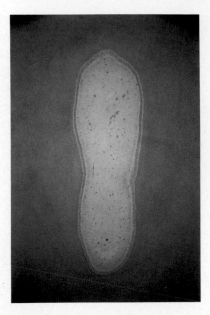

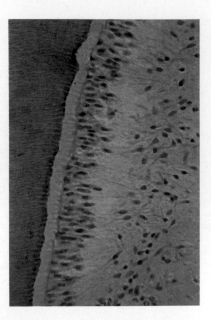

Figure 6–15. Horizontal section of a tooth shows a young pulp tissue enclosed within the dentin. From the light-stained predentin toward the center or core of the pulp are the following pulp zones: odontoblastic, cell-free, and cell-rich. See Fig. 6-16 (at right) for a clear view of the zones in high magnification.

Figure 6–16. This high magnification of the pulp and dentin complex clearly delineates the three pulp zones. The odontoblastic zone is made prominent by its position between the light-stained predentin (left) and the light area of the cell-free zone (right). The cell-rich zone is just to the right of the cell-free zone.

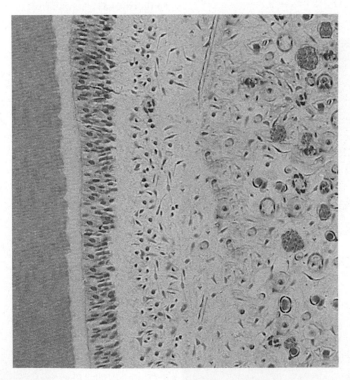

Figure 6–17. Histologic view of the pulp core (right) showing cross sections of larger blood vessels and nerves. Note the density of these structures in the core area in relation to the dentopulpal junction at the left. Can you identify the zones or layers of the pulp?

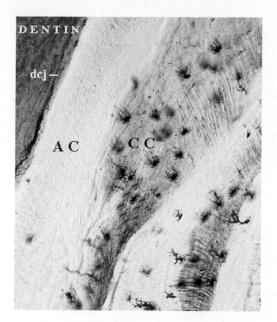

Figure 7–8. Ground section of a root area showing acellular cementum (AC) next to the dentinocemental junction (DCJ) and cellular cementum (CC).

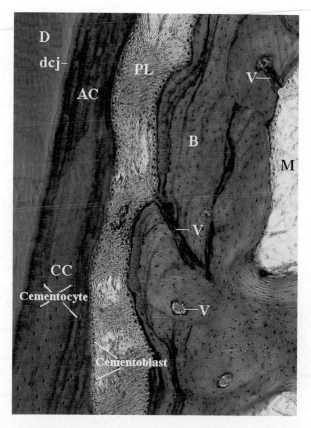

Figure 7–9. Demineralized section of an area of acellular cementum (AC) and cellular cementum (CC). D, dentin; PL, periodontal ligament; B, alveolar bone; DCJ, dentinocemental junction; V, vascular canals; M, bone marrow.

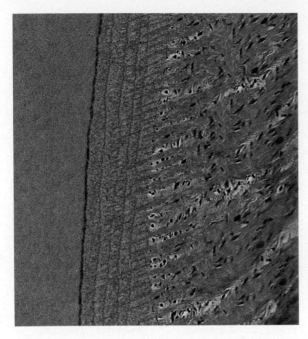

Figure 7–13. Histologic view of root (left) and periodontal ligament (right). Ends of collagen fibers of the periodontal ligament are seen passing into acellular cementum where they are identified as Sharpey's fibers. Note the incremental growth lines running longitudinally within the cementum. The dark-stained line is the dentinocemental junction.

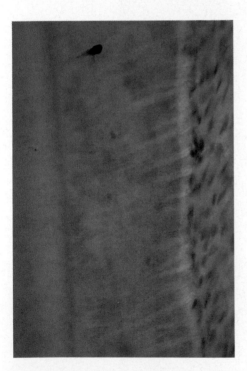

Figure 7–16. Higher magnification of a cellular cementum section with clearly visible Sharpey's fibers. Notice the cementoblast within the periodontal ligament arranged along the lighter-stained cementoid layer and the cementocytes within the cementum.

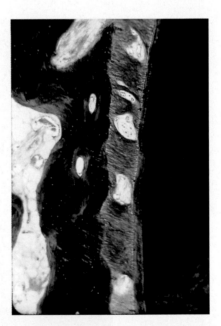

Figure 8–2. Histologic section of an area comparable in position to area X in Fig. 8-1A (p. 174). It was specifically prepared to reveal the arrangement of the collagen fibers of the periodontal ligament between the bone of the socket (left) and the cementum (right). The open areas among the collagen fibers of the periodontal ligament are sites for blood vessels and nerves; the open areas in the bone are sites of bone marrow. Cells were eliminated from the tissues during histologic preparation. See Fig. 8-3 (p. 176) for cellular detail.

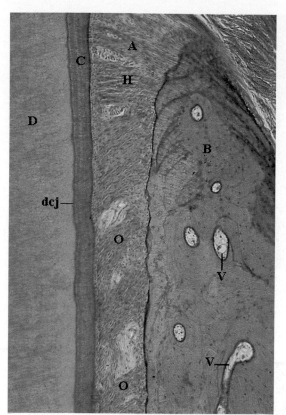

Figure 8–10. Histologic section of the periodontal ligament showing position, direction, and relation of alveolar crest fibers (A), horizontal fibers (H), and oblique fibers (O). C, cementum; D, dentin; DCJ, dentinocemental junction; B, bone (alveolar); V, vascular canals of bone.

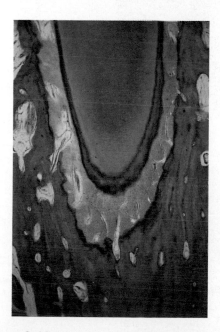

Figure 8–11. Histologic view of the apical part of a tooth, the apical fibers of the periodontal ligament, and the surrounding alveolar bone. Compare the arrangement of the apical fibers shown here to those illustrated in Figs. 8-1 (p. 174) and 8-13 (p. 187).

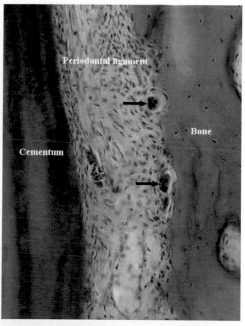

Figure 8–14. (See Color Plate) Photomicrograph of the periodontal ligament between cementum and lamina dura (bone). The arrows indicate two large multinucleate osteoclasts that are in resorption sites along the surface of the lamina dura. Can you identify other cell types? See Figs. 8-5 (p. 178) and 8-13 (p. 187).

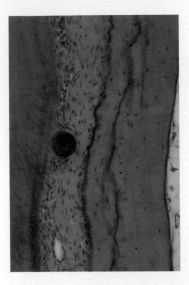

Figure 8–18. Microscopic view of normal-appearing cementum, periodontal ligament, and alveolar bone. Of interest is the cementicle attached to the cementum.

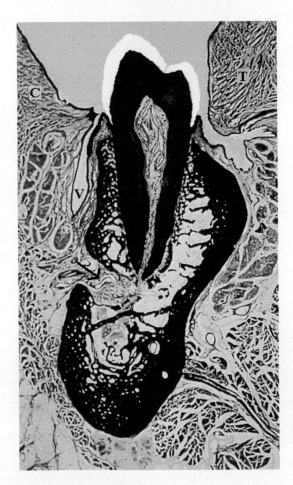

Figure 9–2. Faciolingual section of a human mandible in the region of the second premolar. C, cheek; T, tongue; V, facial vestibule. The arrow is in the mental foramen. How many areas can you identify by referring to Fig. 9-1 (p. 196)?

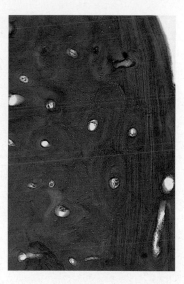

Figure 9–5. Photomicrograph of a demineralized section of compact bone tissue of a human mandible. Cross sections of Haversian systems are present, as are the lacunae that contain cell bodies of osteocytes; circumferential lamellae of the outer surface are also seen (right). See Fig. 9-9 (p. 205) for a diagrammatic interpretation of the vascular canals of compact bone.

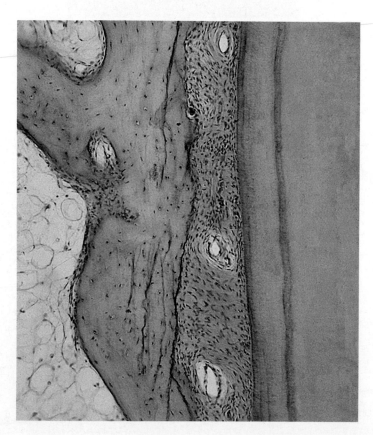

Figure 9–21. From left to right, a microscopic view of the lamina dura (compact bone) of the alveolar process, periodontal ligament, and tooth root. Note the many cells enclosed within both the bone and periodontal ligament in contrast to the obviously acellular cementum. Two sites of yellow bone marrow (fat cells) are present (far left).

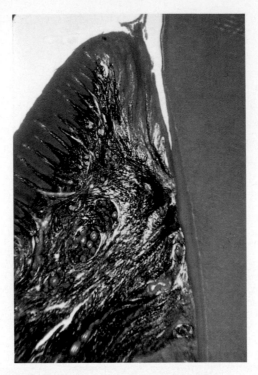

Figure 10–1. Microscopic view of free gingiva adjacent to the cervical part of a tooth. Notice the interdigitation of the surface epithelium with the underlying fibrous connective tissue (lamina propria) and the attachment of the fibers to the cementum.

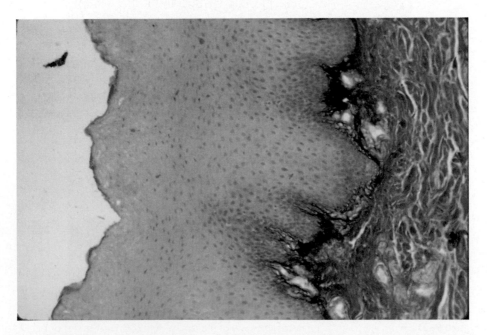

Figure 10–9. Microscopic view of a section of cheek mucosa. Notice the thick epithelial layer and the lack of both a keratin surface layer and the interdigitation of the epithelium and connective tissue. Compare this lining type of oral mucosa to the masticatory type seen in Fig. 10-3 (p. 223).

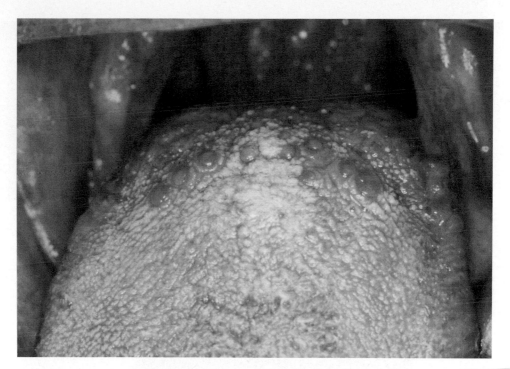

Figure 10–11. Clinical view of the dorsum of the posterior or root of the tongue. Note the large prominent circumvallate papillae arranged in a V pattern. Can you locate the three other types of lingual papillae? See the labels in Fig. 10-10 (p. 229).

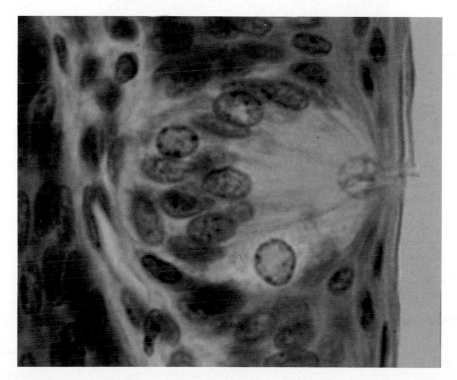

Figure 10–18. Highly magnified view of a taste bud. Note that the taste cells of the bud are arranged like the staves of a barrel and that their nuclei (left) are at the base, opposite to the position of the taste pore at the surface (right).

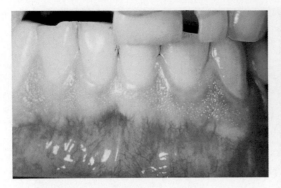

Figure 11–1. Facial side of the anterior mandibular arch. The line between the gingiva and alveolar mucosa is clear. The gingiva is firm, light in color, and stippled in appearance; the interdental papilla fills the interproximal spaces; and the gingival margin can still be observed on the enamel of all teeth. Minute blood vessels are clearly seen in the red, shiny alveolar mucosa.

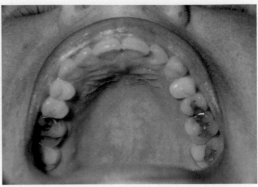

Figure 11–2. Palatal surface of the maxillary arch. The palatal gingiva blends with the mucosa of the hard palate without a line of demarcation. An alveolar mucosa is not present in this area.

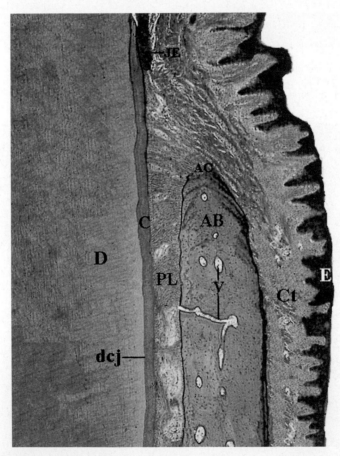

Figure 11–6. Histologic section through a portion of the gingiva and its underlying structures. E, epithelium of the gingiva; CT, connective tissue or lamina propria of the gingiva; AB, alveolar bone; AC, crest of alveolar bone; V, enclosed vascular canals of alveolar bone; PL, periodontal ligament; C, cementum; D, dentin; DCJ, dentinocemental junction; JE, junctional epithelial attachment to the cementum.

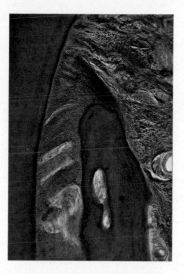

Figure 11–9. Faciolingual histologic section of the mandibular crest region. Note the prominent dentinoperiosteal fibers of the gingiva that pass from the cervical area of the tooth (left), over the crest of the alveolar bone, to the periosteum of the mandibular cortical bone. Dentinogingival and circular fibers are seen above the dentinoperiosteal fibers. Notice the arrangement of periodontal ligament fibers. The section was specially prepared to reveal fibers; cells are not seen.

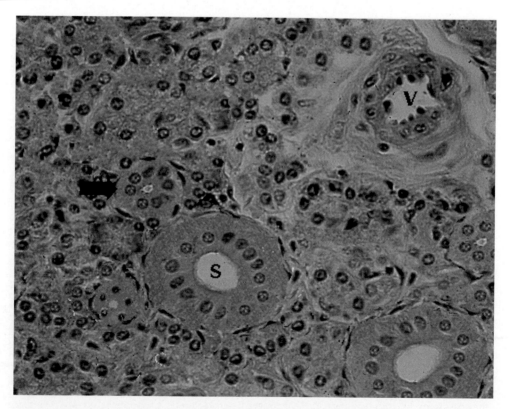

Figure 12–9. High magnification of salivary gland ducts. The arrow points to an intercalated duct. A striated duct lumen (S) and the lumen of a blood vessel (V) are labeled for comparison.

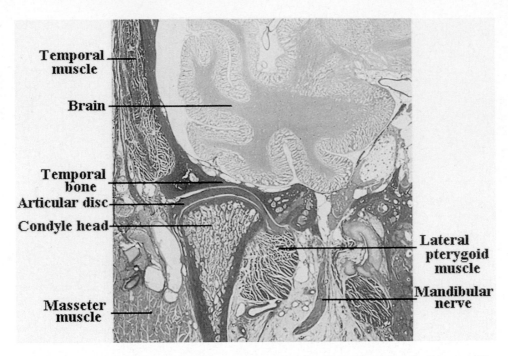

Temporal muscle

Brain

Temporal bone

Articular disc

Condyle head

Lateral pterygoid muscle

Mandibular nerve

Masseter muscle

Figure 14–7. Frontal section through the human temporomandibular joint. Note the thinness of the temporal bone that separates the joint components from the temporal lobe of the brain.

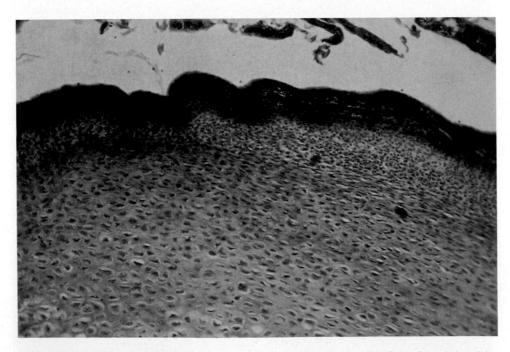

Figure 14–11. Higher magnification of the condylar process seen in Fig. 14-8. Cells of the dark-staining articular surface merge with cells of the underlying hyaline cartilage. Notice that the cells become larger as they pass from the articular surface to the cartilage; this characteristic is appositional growth. The space above the articular surface is the lower joint cavity. Compare with the adult joint in Figs. 14-6 (p. 286) and 14-7 (above).

1 Introduction to Histology

The tissues of the oral cavity are of particular importance in dentistry, and the entire practice of dentistry and dental hygiene is based on knowledge of the structure, arrangement, and reactions of oral tissues to disease. Instructions given to a patient by the dentist and the dental hygienist concerning the correct method of brushing the teeth are based on knowledge of oral histology. A dentist prepares a tooth for a filling with careful attention to the nature and arrangement of the tissues comprising the tooth. The dentist constructs an artificial denture with regard for the structure of the tissues of the palate, alveolar ridge, and oral vestibule. The diseases that occur in the tissues around a tooth when dental plaque or calculus is present can be understood only with a knowledge of tissue structure and tissue reaction, and the tissue repair that follows removal of the calculus can be explained in the same terms. Other diseases of the soft tissues of the mouth are recognized and treated only as normal tissue structure is known. The nearly universal disease of the hard tooth tissues, dental caries, must be described in terms of the microscopic structure of the mineralized tissues of a tooth.

Oral histology is the study of the tissues of the oral cavity: the lining of the mouth and the tissues beneath the lining, the tissues of the tongue, the periodontium, the tooth, the salivary glands, and the tissues from which a tooth develops. This book also includes a study of the process of facial and tooth development.

To understand the oral apparatus, one must have a basic knowledge of how cells are gathered into tissues. The first chapter will summarize the field of general histology and describe the organization of the four basic human tissues: epithelial tissue, connective tissue, muscle tissue, and neural tissue. The relative locations of some of these tissues may be seen in the section through a human mandible at the level of the second premolar tooth (Fig. 1-1).

GENERAL HISTOLOGY

The Nature of Histology

Histology is the science and study of tissues (histo = tissue; logy = science of). This area of anatomy deals with the minute structure, composition, and function of the tissues and is also called *microscopic anatomy*.

A *tissue* is sometimes defined as a grouping of similar cells with intercellular substance and tissue fluid that are combined in a characteristic manner and perform a particular function. Tissues vary greatly in appearance and in structure.

1

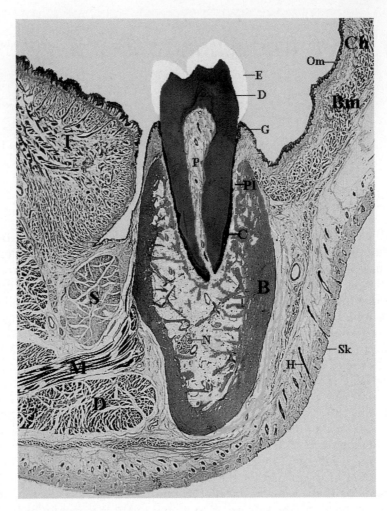

Figure 1–1. (See Color Plates) Photomicrograph of a frontal section through the mandibular second premolar. This picture shows the interdependent relationships among the tissues that make up the components of the oral cavity. Structures derived from epithelial tissue: OM, oral mucosa; G, gingiva; SK, skin; H, hair follicle; S, salivary gland; E, enamel of the tooth. Connective tissue derivatives: B, bone of the mandible; PL, periodontal ligament; CH, connective tissue of the cheek; D, dentin of the tooth; C, cementum of the tooth; P, dental pulp. Muscle tissue derivatives: T, tongue muscles; D, digastric; M, mylohyoid; Bm, buccinator. Nerve tissue derivative: N, inferior alveolar nerve that innervates the teeth, lips, and gums.

Some are hard (bone); some are soft (muscle). Some are sturdy and withstand wear and injury (surface layer of the skin); some are delicate and serve as linings (lining of the respiratory tract). Some are secretory in function (salivary glands); and some are nutritive in function (blood).

HOW TISSUES ARE STUDIED

Microscopic examination of tissues started in the early nineteenth century, and study has been extended and developed as improvements have been made in the construction of microscopes and in the techniques of tissue preparation. Usually, tissues must be stained in some manner to allow their components to be seen clearly with a microscope. Sometimes dyes are injected into the bloodstream of a living animal, and the tissues that have taken up the stain from the blood are subsequently removed from the animal and cut into thin sections. Tissues may be grown in artificial nutrient media in a glass tube, and their growth and development then can be observed from hour to hour or from day to day. Removing a small piece of tissue from the body, embedding it in paraffin, sectioning it, and staining it is the most usual method of tissue preparation.

Let us suppose, for example, that a dentist wants to examine the microscopic structure of the soft tissue surrounding the teeth. A small piece of this gingival tissue is carefully removed from the mouth with a sharp instrument and is immediately placed in a bottle containing a fixative and is sent to a microtechnique laboratory. When the specimen is received in the laboratory, it is dehydrated in absolute alcohol, allowed to stand in xylene, and then placed in a dish of melted paraffin, which is kept in a warming oven. In a few hours, after the paraffin has completely permeated the tissue, they are poured into a small container. Hardened in cool water, the paraffin becomes a firm block that contains the specimen in its center. The paraffin block is then cut into sections (slices) with an instrument called a microtome. In the center of each 8-mm thick section of paraffin is, of course, a section of the embedded specimen. The paraffin sections are arranged on glass microscope slides, with egg albumin used as an adhesive. The slides are then passed through xylene, which dissolves the embedding paraffin, leaving the thin section of tissue attached to the slide. Before the structure of the tissue may be studied, the slides must first be stained appropriately.

The kinds of tissue stains are innumerable. One of the common combinations of stains is hematoxylin and eosin. When the slides bearing the sections of tissue are immersed in the hematoxylin, the nuclei of the cells absorb the stain and become deep blue. Subsequent immersion in the eosin stain causes the cytoplasm of the epithelial cells and the intercellular substance of the connective tissue to become pink. Stains other than hematoxylin and eosin are used to bring out different tissue structures. After the tissue sections are stained, they are covered with a small, thin coverglass. In this way, the slides are permanently preserved.

Specimens that contain mineralized tissue, such as bone and teeth, must be demineralized in a weak acid before they can be cut with the microtome. Demineralization removes (dissolves) the mineral material from the organic material of a tissue and results in certain inevitable changes to tissues. For example, tooth enamel, which is about 96% mineral material and only 4% organic material and water, is usually entirely lost when a tooth is allowed to stand in acid. When the mineral is removed by the acid, the delicate organic portion of the enamel is mechanically washed away unless special techniques for its preservation are employed. Other kinds of mineralized tissues retain their form when they are demineralized. Dentin, cementum, and bone, because they contain a much greater proportion of organic material, are thus not destroyed when the mineral material is removed during demineralization. Completely demineralized dentin, cementum, and bone retain their original shapes but can be easily pierced with a needle.

The enamel of a tooth may be preserved for study if, instead of using the demineralizing, embedding, and sectioning procedures, the tooth is merely ground down to one thin section. This is done on a lathe with a revolving stone. With this technique, one can obtain a tooth section less than 20 microns thick. Specimens of teeth prepared in this way are referred to as *ground sections* (see Frontispiece).

Ground sections are mounted on glass slides and covered with a coverglass in the same way that other types of sections are preserved.

COMPONENTS OF A TISSUE

Tissues are made of *cells, intercellular substance*, and *tissue fluid*. A *cell* is a unit of living substance (protoplasm), and usually consists of cytoplasm and a nucleus. It may exist as an individual, as in unicellular animals, or it may be part of a tissue of a large animal or plant and depend on other cells for existence.

Cells show wide variation in size, shape, and structure. In animals, the largest cell is an ovum, such as a chicken egg or even a human ovum (120 microns in diameter). In contrast to these cells, a human red blood cell is about 8 microns in diameter.

Circulating human red blood cells have lost their nuclei; white blood cells contain one or several nuclei. Muscle cells are distinctive because their cytoplasm has the power of strong contraction. Fat cells contain large amounts of fat, which push the nuclei away from the center of the cells and against the cell walls. The many types of cells, along with the various amounts of intercellular substances and tissue fluid they contain, determine the nature of the various kinds of tissues.

Intercellular substance is a product of living cells and is distributed among the cells in all the tissues of the body. It holds the cells together and provides a medium for the passage of nutrients and waste materials from capillaries to cells and from cells to capillaries. The amount and kind of intercellular substance differ among tissues. In some human tissues, such as bone, intercellular substance is the predominant element, whereas other tissues, such as the epithelium that makes up the surface of the skin, contain less intercellular substance and cellular elements predominate. Intercellular substance occurs in two forms: One form is *fibrous* in nature and the other is *amorphous* in nature (a = without; morphous = form) (Fig. 1-2).

The fibrous part of the intercellular substance is formed by cells of the tissue and referred to as *formed elements*. Four types of these fibrous or formed elements are found in the human body—*collagen, reticulum, elastic*, and *oxytalan*. Reticulum fibers are considered to be younger forms of collagen fibers, and oxytalan fibers younger forms of elastic fibers.

The amorphous part of the intercellular substance is commonly referred to as *ground substance*. It functions as a molecular sieve, allowing the passage of metabolites between the blood and tissues, and also serves as a physical barrier to prevent the spread of foreign elements, such as microorganisms. The ground substance is a complex of chemical substances known as mucopolysaccharides (also called *glycosaminoglycans* and *proteoglycans*). Students who are interested in the structural, physical, and chemical features of the fibrous and ground substance types of intercellular substance should consult standard general histology textbooks.

Tissue fluid is the part of the blood plasma that can diffuse through the walls of capillaries. In the tissue, fluid nutrients are carried out through capillary walls to the surrounding intercellular substance and then to the cells; waste products of the cells are returned in the same manner from the intercellular substance to the capillaries. Tissue fluid may be present in a tissue in relatively small proportions, as in

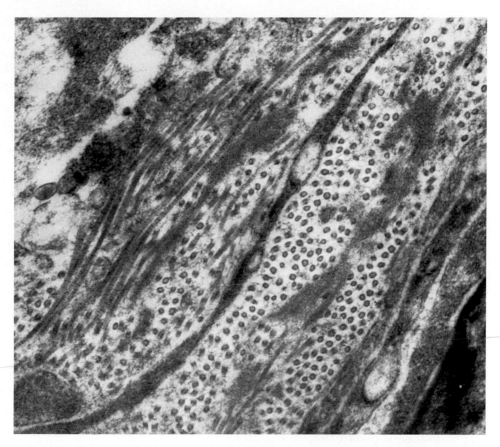

Figure 1–2. Electron micrograph of connective tissue shows the two forms of intercellular substance. The fibrous form is collagen fibrils cut in cross and longitudinal sections. The longitudinally cut fibrils, running diagonally from top to bottom on the left side, reveal cross-banding, a characteristic of collagen fibrils. The amorphous or ground substance is seen as clear areas around the collagen fibrils. (Courtesy of Dr. Dennis Foreman.)

the epithelium of the surface of the skin, or it may form a large proportion of the tissue, as in blood. The tissue fluid of epithelium, bone, and other tissue is, of course, derived from blood.

CLASSIFICATION OF TISSUES

In their function and gross and microscopic appearance, tissues vary so widely that the beginning student may recognize little or no relationship among them. This seeming confusion lessens, however, when the student discovers that, for purposes of easier study and better understanding, histologists have developed a classification for tissues. Tissues are alike in that they are made of cells, intercellular substance, and tissue fluid. Tissues differ in the form and number of cells, in the type and amount of intercellular substance, and in the amount of tissue fluid. These similarities and differences among tissues are the bases that histologists have used to develop a classification of tissues.

Human tissues have been assorted into *four primary groups*: *epithelial tissue*, *connective tissue*, *muscle tissue*, and *nerve tissue*. The tissues of each of these primary groups share certain fundamental characteristics, but because differences also exist within the groups, each of the four primary groups has been subdivided. The subdivisions are based on structural differences that clearly distinguish one tissue from another.

A brief classification of human tissues is presented in Table 1-1.

Tissues are combined in characteristic ways to form *organs*, such as the heart, lungs, liver, bones, skin, and tongue, and organs are combined in characteristic ways to form *organisms*, such as the human body.

Let us consider the tongue as an organ. The tongue is made of a combination of each of the four basic tissues: epithelial tissue, connective tissue, muscle tissue, and nerve tissue, all of which are interdependent in the functioning organ (Fig. 1-3). Epithelial tissue comprises the surface of the tongue and serves as a protective covering; within the tongue is another type of epithelial tissue in the form of several sizable salivary glands. Beneath the surface epithelium is connective tissue, which supplies both support and nourishment; beneath this layer of connective tissue are strong muscles that produce the organ's movement. Nerves of the tongue supply both motor and sensory functions.

Another organ of the human body is the skin. Skin is made of a combination of epithelial tissue, connective tissue, and nerves. The skin covers and protects other body organs, such as bones and muscles. Bones support the body, and muscles move the bones and other organs under the direction of the nervous system, which supplies the impulses. The entire organism is nourished by blood pumped through the pipeline of the blood vessels by the cardiac muscle, which is the chief tissue of the heart. The next sections will review the characteristics of each of the four basic tissues.

Table I–I. Classification of Tissues

Epithelial Tissue
    Surface cells of covering and lining membranes (e.g., skin of mucous membranes)
    Glandular tissue

Connective Tissue
    Fibrous (e.g., skin beneath the epithelium)
    Loose areolar (e.g., thin membranes between various layers of tissue)
    Adipose (fat)
    Hemopoietic (i.e., bone marrow and lymphatic tissue)
    Cartilage
    Bone

Nerve Tissue
    Tissue of central nervous system
    Tissue of peripheral nervous system

Muscle Tissue
    Smooth involuntary (e.g., wall of intestines)
    Striated voluntary (skeletal muscle)
    Striated involuntary (heart muscle)

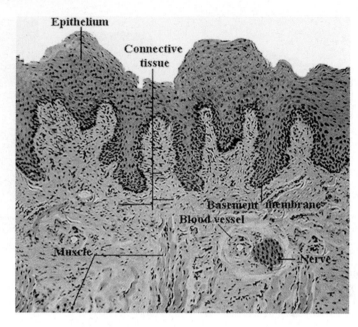

Figure 1–3. Histologic section through a human tongue showing the interrelationship among the four basic tissues.

EPITHELIAL TISSUE

Epithelial tissue is distributed widely throughout the body and has many different kinds of structure. It occurs as a covering or lining tissue, such as the surface layer of the skin and the surface layer of the mucous membranes, which line body cavities such as the mouth, stomach, and intestines. Epithelial tissue also gives rise to several organs during embryonic development, such as the highly specialized cells of the pancreas, liver, thyroid gland, and salivary glands. In addition, in certain locations in the upper and lower jaws, epithelial tissue becomes differentiated into structures called the *enamel organs*, which are located deep in the jaw and produce the enamel of developing teeth (see Chapter 3). Although the various kinds of epithelial tissues all have a proportionally large number of cells and little intercellular substance, their structure in different locations in the body is adapted to the functions they perform.

All lining and glandular epithelial tissues rest on a connective tissue. Interposed between the epithelial and connective tissues is a structure called the *basement membrane* (Figs. 1-3 and 1-4). Viewed under a light microscope, the basement membrane appears as a single layer. Electron microscopic views, however, reveal that the basement membrane is actually composed of two layers, or *laminae*, that are composed of fibers and ground substance. The *basal lamina* is secreted by the adjacent epithelial cells and comprised mostly of ground substance, and the *reticular lamina* is produced by cells of the connective tissue and is more fibrous.

The basement membrane serves several functions: It supports and cushions the epithelium; it connects the epithelium to the connective tissue; and it acts as a filtration barrier for both the epithelium and the connective tissue.

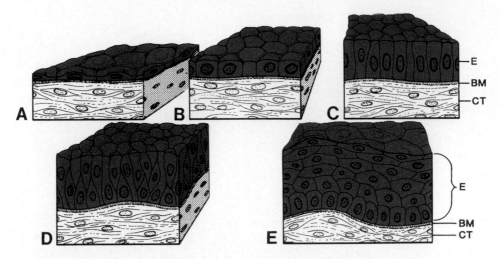

Figure 1–4. Diagrammatic drawings of different types of lining epithelia. The epithelium (E) is connected to the underlying connective tissue (CT) by a basement membrane (BM). **A.** Simple squamous epithelium. **B.** Simple cuboidal epithelium. **C.** Simple columnar epithelium. **D.** Pseudostratified columnar epithelium. **E.** Stratified squamous epithelium.

For purposes of description, histologists have classified epithelial tissues into two major groups and several subgroups:

    I.   Surface cells of covering and lining membranes
        A. Simple
            1. Squamous
            2. Cuboidal
            3. Columnar
        B. Pseudostratified columnar
        C. Stratified
            1. Squamous
            2. Cuboidal
            3. Columnar
            4. Transitional
   II. Glandular tissue
        A. Endocrine glands (e.g., thyroid)
        B. Exocrine glands (e.g., salivary glands)
        C. Mixed endocrine and exocrine (e.g., pancreas)

SURFACE EPITHELIA

Epithelial cells of covering and lining membranes are not all alike in shape and arrangement. The shape of epithelial cells is described by the words squamous, cuboidal, and columnar; the arrangement of epithelial cells is described by the words simple, stratified, and pseudostratified. The word *squamous* means scale-like or flat, and *squamous epithelial cells* are flat cells. *Cuboidal epithelial cells* are roughly cube shaped, and *columnar epithelial cells* are tall and narrow. When the arrangement of epithelial cells is in a single layer, the tissue is said to be *simple ep-*

ithelium. When epithelial cells are arranged in several layers, the tissue is called *stratified epithelium* (stratified = in layers). The word *pseudostratified* is applied to an arrangement of columnar epithelial cells in which the cells appear to be stratified but are actually in a single layer (pseudo = false).

All simple epithelia are delicate in structure and found only in areas of the body that are subjected to little or no friction in functional use. *Simple squamous epithelium* (a single layer of flat epithelial cells) lines the inside of the walls of blood vessels (Fig. 1-4A). *Simple cuboidal epithelium* (a single layer of cuboidal epithelial cells) is in the covering epithelium of the ovary (Fig. 1-4B). *Simple columnar epithelium* (a single layer of columnar epithelial cells) lines the cervix of the uterus (Fig. 1-4C).

Pseudostratified columnar epithelium (Fig. 1-4D) makes up the epithelial part of the mucous membrane that lines the upper respiratory tract: the maxillary sinuses, the nasal cavity, and the trachea. This epithelium is actually composed of a single layer of columnar epithelial cells. However, because the nucleus is located near the base of some cells, whereas in other cells the nucleus is located nearer the outer end, this epithelium has the appearance of being made of two or three layers of cells. In the upper respiratory tract, the pseudostratified columnar epithelium is supplied with *cilia* and *goblet cells*. Cilia are minute, hair-like projections that cover the surface ends of the columnar cells and act as dust catchers or filters for the air breathed in through the nose. Goblet cells are modified epithelial cells that are interspersed among the other columnar cells and secrete substances that keep the tissue surface of the nose and sinuses moist.

Stratified epithelium consists of cells that are similar in shape to cells of simple epithelium, but that are arranged from two to three layers in depth. *Stratified cuboidal epithelium* and *stratified columnar epithelium* occur as the lining of some of the larger ducts of glands, such as the large ducts of the major salivary glands. The stratified epithelial cells that line the urinary bladder change in shape from round to flat, depending on whether the bladder is empty or full; this epithelium is therefore described as *stratified transitional epithelium*. Stratified epithelium is more resistant to hard use than are the simple types of epithelium. By far the most sturdy of all kinds of epithelia is *stratified squamous epithelium*, which covers all surfaces of the body that are routinely subjected to considerable wear and tear.

Stratified squamous epithelium (Figs. 1-3 and 1-4E) makes up both the surface of the skin and the surface of the mucous membrane of the oral cavity. In both of these locations, the epithelium is composed of many layers of cells and, as is true with all epithelia, rests on the *basement membrane*, which separates the epithelial tissue from its underlying connective tissue. The epithelial cells of the deepest layer, called *basal cells*, are not flat but are somewhat cuboidal and often show cell division. As these basal cells multiply, some cells are gradually moved toward the outside surface, becoming flatter as they approach the surface and finally becoming dead cells. In some areas of the oral cavity, the flat, dead epithelial cells on the surface are sloughed off as they are replaced from below. In other areas of the oral cavity and on the skin, these dead surface cells are not quickly sloughed off. Instead they may lose their nuclei and cell boundaries and become converted into a tough, resistant surface layer, which is called the *keratinized layer* (Fig. 1-5). This keratinized layer gradually wears off and is replaced from beneath as a result of continued cell division in the basal cell layer. The most heavily keratinized epithelium of the body is found on the palms of the hands and on the soles of the feet (Fig. 1-6), particularly if these areas have been subjected to hard use and are calloused.

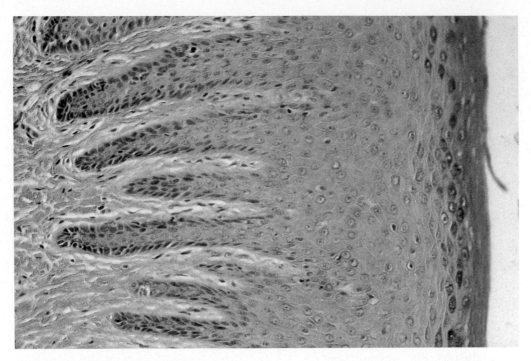

Figure 1–5. (See Color Plates) Photomicrograph of an oral mucous membrane section. A darker-stained stratified squamous epithelium is interdigitating with and connected to an underlying lighter-stained fibrous connective tissue. The surface layer of the epithelium is keratin. Compare to Figs. 1-2 and 1-6.

Nonkeratinized and keratinized epithelium are described further in the study of the oral mucosa (see Chapter 10).

Covering and lining epithelial tissues do not contain blood vessels; they receive nourishment via the blood vessels contained in the connective tissue that surrounds or underlies them.

GLANDULAR TISSUE

Glands are secreting organs that produce a specific product or secretion. The parenchyma or secretory component of a gland is derived from epithelial tissue. These epithelial cells are specialized to produce secretions.

Glands can be classified in several ways. No attempt is made here to deal with them all, but those that are more commonly used are reviewed in general terms. The interested student should consult any of the many fine general histology textbooks for further information.

During development, all glands arise as an invagination of covering or lining epithelium into the underlying connective tissue or stroma. The epithelium, at first, is a solid mass of cells. These epithelial cells continue to proliferate and migrate, and become the glandular epithelium that eventually gives rise to all epithelial portions of the gland.

The surface connection may remain intact, thus retaining a union between the secretory epithelial cells and the free surface (e.g., surface of skin and of oral cavity). Eventually the epithelium hollows out throughout its length, providing a transport duct system for the secretions. This type of gland is classified as a duct gland. Because the secretion of this type of gland is discharged onto the surface from which it developed, it is also classified as an *exocrine* gland (gland of external secretion).

The continuous invaginated glandular epithelium of some developing glands may lose the connection with the free surface, and the secretory epithelial cells consequently become isolated from the site of origin. Because this type of gland loses the transport system to a free surface, it is called a *ductless* gland. The secretions of this type of gland diffuse into the nearby blood and lymph vessels. Because it discharges its products internally, it is also called an *endocrine* gland.

The glands can be classified according to the kind of secretion they produce. Endocrine (ductless) glands secrete hormones. Hormones are chemical substances secreted into blood and lymph vessels and have specific effects on the activities of other cells and organs.

Secretions produced by exocrine glands may be *serous, mucous*, or a combination of serous and mucous. The secretory cells of these glands are named according to the type of secretion they produce (e.g., serous or mucous cells). If a particular

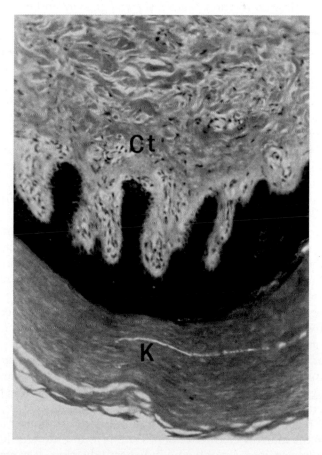

Figure 1–6. Histologic section of the sole of a human foot. K, heavily keratinized surface layer of the epithelium; CT, underlying connective tissue. Compare this section of skin to the section of oral mucous membrane seen in Fig. 1-5.

gland is composed of only serous cells, it is referred to as a pure serous gland; if a gland is composed of only mucous cells, it is referred to as a pure mucous gland. *Mixed* glands have both serous and mucous cells making their secretory portions, and their products are described as *seromucous* secretions.

In summary, some glands are classified as exocrine because their ducts open onto the external surface of the body (e.g., see discussion of salivary glands in Chapter 12). Other glands are classified as endocrine or ductless because their secretions enter the blood as hormones.

CONNECTIVE TISSUE

Connective tissues are comprised of a relatively larger amount of intercellular substance and relatively fewer cells than are epithelial cells. In spite of this characteristic, connective tissues differ so greatly in form and function that at first glance they sometimes appear to be unrelated to one another. Fibrous connective tissue underlies the epithelium of the skin and oral mucosa and makes up tendons and ligaments. Areolar connective tissue attaches skin to muscle; fat connective tissue stores food; hemopoietic connective tissue forms blood. Cartilage connective tissue provides support and permits skeletal growth, and bone connective tissue supports the body.

Fibrous connective tissue is found throughout the body. In its most dense form, it makes up tendons and ligaments; in a less dense form, it underlies the epithelial part of skin and mucous membranes (Figs. 1-1, 1-2, 1-3, 1-5, and 1-6). Like other tissue, fibrous connective tissue is made of cells and intercellular substance. There are two kinds of intercellular substance—fibrillar and amorphous ground substance. The fibrillar component of intercellular substance is the predominant element.

The fibers of fibrous connective tissue are made of minute fibrils and produced by cells called *fibroblasts* (blast = germ, builder). Special staining techniques used on histologic sections reveal that the fibers are not all alike: Some are *collagenous fibers*; others are *elastic fibers*. These fibers are distributed in different proportions in different kinds of fibrous connective tissue.

Suspended with the fibers in the all-encompassing amorphous ground substance are the various kinds of cells of the fibrous connective tissue. Proportionally, the most numerous cells are the *fibroblasts*. Special tissue preparations also reveal the presence of other types of cells, some of which are capable of becoming defense cells when the tissue suffers injury or bacterial infection.

Areolar connective tissue is seen during any gross dissection of a mammal in which skin is attached to muscles, muscles are attached to muscles, or internal organs are held together by membranes of connective tissue. These tissue membranes, called *fascia*, are made of areolar connective tissue and fat tissue. The areolar connective tissue is composed of a relatively small number of cells and a loose, thin network of fibrous intercellular substance, all held together by a large amount of ground substance.

Fat tissue (Fig. 1-7) is distributed throughout the body among the soft tissues and in the marrow cavities of bones and is found more or less generously concentrated in certain parts of the body beneath the skin. It is composed of specialized connective tissue cells, called *fat cells*, which are held together by fibrous intercellular substance and are capable of storing fat. They may become so filled with fat

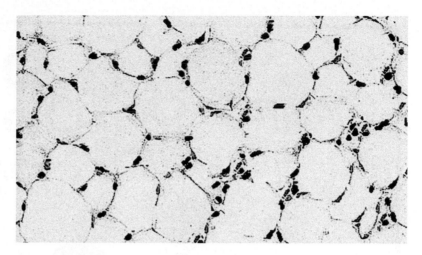

Figure 1–7. Histologic section of a fatty type of connective tissue. Fat is stored in the ringed areas. Fat nuclei are pushed to the periphery of the rings; at this magnification, the cell nuclei resemble dots.

that the cytoplasm is pressed into a thin layer around the periphery of the cell and the nucleus is crowded against the side of the cell.

Hemopoietic tissue (hemo = blood; poietic = to make) not only produces blood cells that are added to the circulating blood, but also removes worn out blood cells from the bloodstream. In adults, hemopoietic tissue occurs in two different forms, as *red bone marrow* and as *lymphatic tissue*. In the human fetus, red bone marrow is found in nearly all the bones, but in the adult, the marrow in many of the bones has become converted to so-called *yellow bone marrow*, which is largely fat. Certain bones, however, such as the vault of the skull, the ribs, the sternum, and the bodies of vertebrae, retain the red bone marrow throughout adult life. Yellow bone marrow in other bones can be converted into hemopoietic red marrow in circumstances of emergency.

Red bone marrow consists of a fibrillar meshwork of intercellular substance throughout which are scattered many cells that have the potential to differentiate into several kinds of blood cells. Red bone marrow produces *red bone cells* (*erythrocytes*) and certain kinds of *white blood cells* (*granular leukocytes*), which are white blood cells that have granules in the cytoplasm (*eosinophilic leukocytes*, *basophilic leukocytes*, and *neutrophilic leukocytes*) (Fig. 1-8).

Lymphatic tissue is composed of fibrillar intercellular substance and scattered undifferentiated cells. Some of these undifferentiated cells are capable of becoming differentiated into certain kinds of white blood cells, chiefly *lymphocytes*. Conspicuous areas of lymphatic tissue are seen in several places around the oral cavity: the palatine tonsils located between the oral cavity and the pharynx, and the lingual tonsils located on the posterior part of the dorsum of the tongue. Lymphatic tissue is found also in other parts of the body.

In *cartilage* (Fig. 1-9), the most conspicuous component of the tissue is the ground substance type of intercellular substance, which in gross examination resembles a firm gel. Fibers, which may be made visible by special histologic preparation of tissue sections, are scattered throughout the ground substance. The cells of cartilage, called *chondrocytes*, occupy spaces, called *lacunae*, in the intercellular

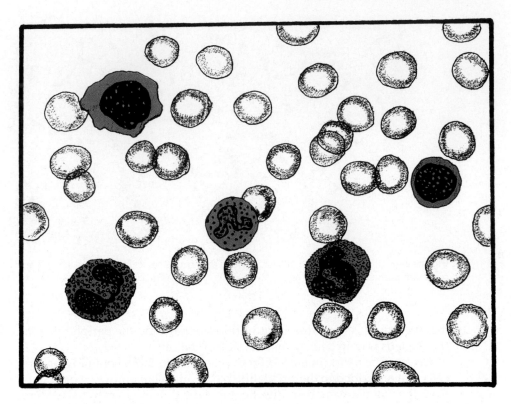

Figure 1–8. Diagrammatic illustration of a human blood smear. The more numerous red blood cells (erythrocytes) are small biconcave disks about 8 microns in diameter that have neither a nucleus nor cytoplasmic granules. The five larger cells (highlighted) are different types of white blood cells (leukocytes), which have nuclei; some have granules in the cytoplasm. The nongranular leukocytes are the large lymphocyte (upper left) and the small lymphocyte (upper right), which have round nuclei. The three white blood cells below are granular leukocytes, which have multilobed nuclei and conspicuous cytoplasmic granules. From left to right, these cells are an eosinophilic leukocyte, a basophilic leukocyte, and a neutrophilic leukocyte.

substance. Nutrients are transmitted to the cells through the intercellular substance. Cartilage exists as a nonmineralized tissue.

A large part of the skeleton of the human fetus is first constructed in cartilage, which seems to act as a pattern for the developing bone tissue. The arm and leg bones, for example, are first formed in cartilage, which is resorbed as bone tissue develops to replace it (see Chapter 9). Whereas bone replaces most cartilage in the human skeleton at an early stage, cartilage persists in some places for years. At the ends of the long bones, the presence of cartilage throughout childhood and adolescence permits the bones to grow in length. In adults, cartilage comprises parts of the nose, larynx, trachea, and ear. Cartilage tissue contains no nerves or blood vessels.

Bone is mineralized connective tissue (Fig. 1-10) and contains a large amount of dense fibrous intercellular substance. The fibrils that make up the fibrous intercellular substance are surrounded by ground substance, in which mineral salts are deposited in solution as the bone is developing. As the bone matures, these mineral salts crystallize out of solution, and the bone becomes a mineralized tissue.

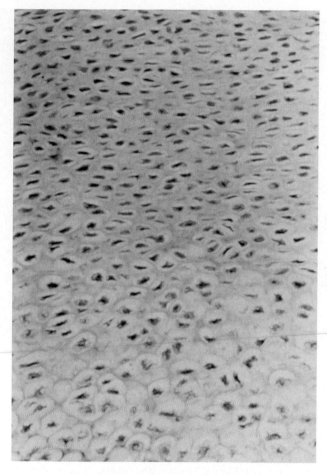

Figure 1–9. Histologic section of a type of cartilage. The cells (chondrocytes) are in lacunae. The variation in chondrocyte size indicates stages of growth within the cartilage skeleton.

The cells of bone, called *osteocytes*, occupy lacunae in the hard intercellular substance. Chapter 9 includes more about the microscopic picture of bone tissue.

A type of connective tissue with which you will become familiar in subsequent chapters is embryonic or young connective tissue called *mesenchyme*.[1] Cells or tissues that arise from this type of tissue are *mesenchymal* in origin. For instance, the cells that form dentin and cementum of a tooth are connective tissue cells that arise from mesenchymal tissues; the dental pulp tissue is a mature mesenchymal tissue.

NERVE TISSUE

Nerve tissue, which comprises the entire nervous system, is made of nerve cells and the neuroglial cells that support them. Nerve cells are called *neurons*. Although, like other cells, they have a nucleus and a cytoplasm, they also are highly specialized and differ from other cells. Neurons can react to stimuli (i.e., they are

---

[1] Mesenchyme (pronounced *měs' ĕn kĭm*) is an embryonic connective tissue. The adjective is mesenchymal (*měs ĕn' kĭm al*).

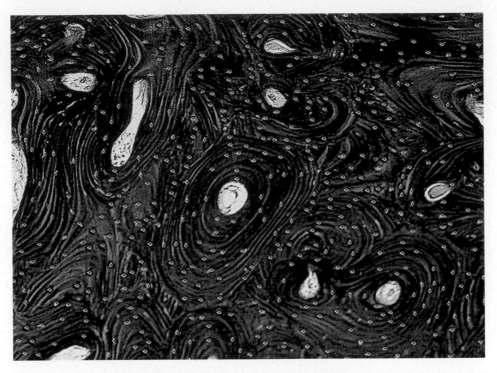

Figure 1–10. Microscopic view of human compact bone tissue. The bone-forming cells (osteocytes) are located in lacunae (small spaces). The larger spaces (Haversian canals) represent the vascular channels of the bone. Notice how the bone is formed in concentric rings around the central canal.

irritable) and transmit waves of excitation from the point at which a stimulus is applied (i.e., they can conduct impulses). These waves of excitation, or *nerve impulses*, are transmitted along the cell membrane of the neuron, which is peculiarly adapted to this function.

The nervous system consists of two chief divisions: The *central nervous system* (the brain and spinal cord) and the *peripheral nervous system* (nerves associated with the various other organs of the body). The gross appearance and histologic structure of the nerve tissue are different in these two divisions. The tissue of the central nervous system is extremely soft because of the absence of connective tissue as a supporting tissue for the nerve cells. In the central nervous system, nerve cells are supported by a specialized cell population called *neuroglia* (neuro = nerve, glia = glue). The brain and spinal cord are made of two distinct types of this soft nerve tissue, called *gray matter* and *white matter*, that differ greatly in histologic structure.

In contrast to the nerve tissue of the central nervous system, nerves of the peripheral nervous system are tough. This firm quality is derived from the considerable amount of connective tissue that covers and supports the bundles of nerve fibers. A microscopic examination of a cross section of a nerve reveals that it is circular and is covered by a connective tissue wrapping, or sheath. Inside this sheath are several bundles of *nerve fibers*; each bundle is surrounded by another connective tissue sheath. Each nerve fiber inside the bundles is encased in its individual connective tissue sheath, and often between this sheath and the individual fiber is

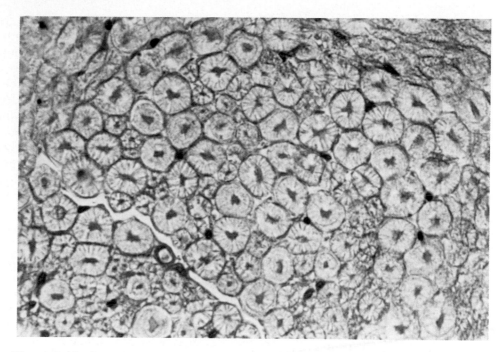

Figure 1–11. Cross section of a myelinated peripheral nerve. Shrunken axons appear as dark spots surrounded by a myelin sheath.

a layer of substance of a fatty nature called a *myelin sheath* (Fig. 1-11). Each nerve fiber in this nerve is actually a long, thin, stretched-out part of the cytoplasm of a neuron. The body of the neuron, which contains the nucleus, lies deep in the body of the individual.

Nerve cells do not multiply with the growth of the human body. A person is born with all the neurons he or she will possess. If a fiber in the peripheral nervous system is cut, however, repair may eventually take place. The end of the fiber that has been cut off degenerates, and the part of the fiber still attached to the body of the neuron may grow to the length of the original fiber. In the central nervous system, on the other hand, damage is permanent. No regeneration follows damage to the brain or spinal cord.

MUSCLE TISSUE

Muscle tissue is composed of muscle cells that are supported by connective tissue. Muscle cells are much longer than they are wide, and for this reason an individual muscle cell is called a muscle fiber. Muscle fibers have the property of contraction to a degree greater than that of other cells.

Microscopic examination of muscle tissue from various parts of the body reveals a difference in the appearance of the cytoplasm of muscle fibers. In muscle tissue from some areas, such as from the intestine, the cytoplasm of the muscle fibers appears relatively clear. In muscle tissue from other areas, such as from the arm or heart, the cytoplasm of the muscle fibers has cross striations. This difference in the appearance of the cytoplasm of different muscle fibers led histologists to classify muscle tissue as *smooth muscle tissue* (in which the cytoplasm of the fibers is not cross striated) and *striated muscle tissue* (in which the cytoplasm of the fibers is cross striated).

This division of muscle tissue into two types was not quite adequate, however. Smooth muscle is *involuntary muscle*, and the contraction of its fibers is not under the control of the individual. For instance, the peristaltic movements of the intestine, which contains smooth muscle in its walls, are not willfully controlled. On the other hand, striated muscle is for the most part *voluntary muscle* because the contractions of the muscle fibers may be consciously controlled by the individual. One moves an arm or a leg as one wishes. However, although the fibers of the heart muscle are striated like the fibers of the muscles of the arm, they are not consciously controlled by the individual. Therefore, cardiac muscle has been assigned to its own class, called *striated involuntary muscle*, in contrast to skeletal muscle, which is referred to as *striated voluntary muscle*.

Thus, a classification for muscle tissue consists of three categories: *smooth muscle*, *striated voluntary muscle*, and *striated involuntary muscle* (Fig. 1-12).

Smooth muscle tissue is found in such places as the walls of the intestines, the blood vessels, and the roots of hairs, where its contraction produces an erection of the hair. The individual muscle fibers (cells) of smooth muscle tissue are shaped somewhat like a cigar and have a centrally located nucleus. They may vary in length from 1/1000 mm in the small blood vessels to 1/2 mm in the pregnant uterus. The fibers are supported by associated connective tissue.

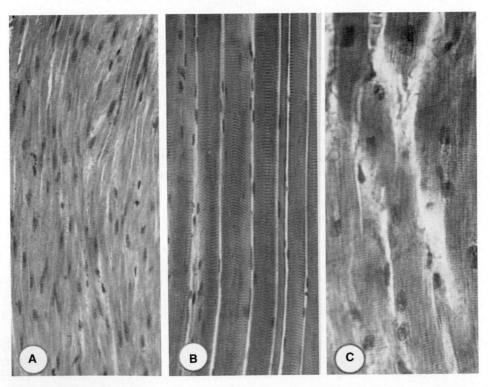

Figure 1–12. Sections of muscle types. **A.** Smooth muscle. **B.** Striated voluntary muscle. **C.** Striated involuntary muscle (cardiac) with intercalated discs.

Striated voluntary muscle is known also as *skeletal muscle*. As well as the obvious inclusion in this class of muscles such as those that move the arms and legs, skeletal muscles also include those in and about the oral cavity—muscles of the tongue, lips and cheeks, and soft palate. The muscle fibers of skeletal muscle differ in several ways from those of smooth muscle. The difference in the appearance of the cytoplasm, which shows microscopic cross striations (Fig. 1-12), is most conspicuous. In addition, the nuclei in skeletal muscle fibers are pushed to one side of the fibers instead of lying in the center, and a fiber may contain more than one nucleus. Skeletal muscle fibers are relatively long, varying from 1 to 40 mm, and are supported by connective tissue that covers individual fibers and binds them into bundles. This supporting connective tissue is well supplied with blood vessels and nerves.

Striated involuntary muscle is confined to the heart and is known as *cardiac muscle*. Although its microscopic appearance resembles skeletal muscle in that the cytoplasm of the muscle fibers contain microscopic cross striations (Fig. 1-12), the fibers are arranged differently. Whereas skeletal muscle fibers exist as individual fibers with several nuclei, cardiac muscle fibers branch and come together so that they form a sort of network that comprises the heart muscle. This network is supported by surrounding connective tissue that contains nerves and a rich supply of blood vessels.

Muscles are the organs responsible for both the voluntary and the involuntary movement of all the parts of the body. They act in response to impulses received from the nervous system and are surrounded, supported, and nourished by the connective tissues (fibrous, areolar, and adipose), bones, cartilage, and blood.

ORAL HISTOLOGY

The structures of the oral cavity are derived from the four basic tissues described above. The mucous membranes of the mouth and the salivary gland are derived from epithelial tissue. The bone of the jaw and the fibers of periodontal ligament originate from connective tissue. The muscles attached to the mandible and which form the core of the tongue are derived from muscle tissue. Finally, the nerves that innervate the oral cavity are derivatives of nervous tissue.

TISSUES OF A TOOTH

Although the oral cavity is composed of the same basic tissues as the rest of the body, there are specializations unique to this area. Specifically, the tissues that make up tooth are derivatives of epithelial and connective tissues. Figures 1-13 and 1-14 are diagrams of teeth that have been cut approximately through the middle in a faciolingual direction to depict the relationship between the enamel, dentin, pulp, and cementum. *Tooth enamel* comprises the surface of the crown of the tooth and is derived from epithelial cells. In contrast, dentin, pulp, and cementum all originate from connective tissue cells.

The line of union between the epithelial-derived enamel and the connective tissue–derived dentin is the *dentinoenamel junction*; the line of union between the

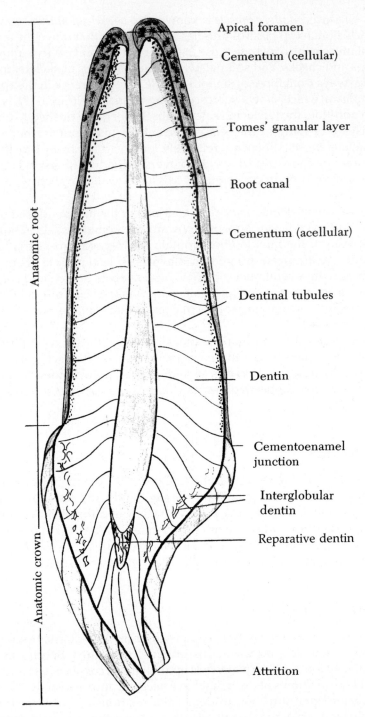

Figure I–I3. Diagrammatic drawing of a longitudinal faciolingual section of a maxillary incisor. The cementum lacunae in this diagram and in Fig. 1-14 are somewhat exaggerated in size.

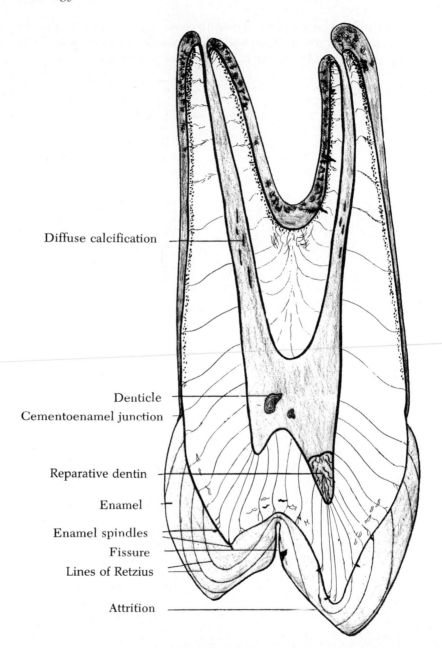

Diffuse calcification

Denticle

Cementoenamel junction

Reparative dentin

Enamel

Enamel spindles

Fissure

Lines of Retzius

Attrition

Figure 1–14. Diagrammatic drawing of a longitudinal faciolingual section of a maxillary first premolar. See Frontispiece for a photograph of a similar tooth, and compare the structures indicated in this diagrammatic drawing with the same structures seen in the photograph of an actual tooth section.

dentin and the cementum is the *dentinocemental junction*. The line of union between the cementum and the enamel is the *cementoenamel junction*. These junctions are frequent points of reference in descriptions of a tooth.

SUGGESTED READING

Gartner LP, Hiatt JL, Strum JM. Cell Biology and Histology. 2nd Ed. Philadelphia: Lippincott Williams & Wilkins, 1997.

2 Embryonic Development of the Face and Oral Cavity

THE HUMAN BODY

The Beginning of a Human Body

Beginning of life for an individual human being is the moment the sperm unites with the ovum and forms a fertilized egg. The fertilized egg is called a *zygote* (zygotus = yoked together). This egg divides into two cells, each of these into two more, and the resulting cells divide again and again. At first, only a mass of slightly differentiated cells exists; then shaping begins—a shaping that eventually results in the formation of a tiny tubular embryo that foreshadows the plan of the adult human body.

An adult body is essentially a thick-walled tube. Or, perhaps it can be better described as two tubes, a larger outer tube (outside body wall) and a smaller inner tube (digestive tract), between which is a space (body cavity) that contains the internal organs: heart, lungs, liver. The mouth is the *cephalic* (head) opening of the inner tube, and the anus is the *caudal* (tail) opening.

In the tiny embryo, the tube that is the outside body wall also encases a smaller tube, the *primitive digestive tract*, or *primitive gut*, which, at this time, is closed at both ends because the mouth and anus have not yet formed. In early stages of development, before the internal organs are formed, cells located between the outer body wall and the primitive digestive tract make the wall of the tubular embryo relatively thick.

The embryonic body wall is made of three layers: *ectoderm* (ecto = outside; derm = skin), *mesoderm* (meso = middle), and *endoderm* (endo = inside). Collectively, these layers are called *primary embryonic layers*, or *primary germ layers*, and each is destined to form certain organs, or parts of organs, of the adult body. For example, ectoderm gives rise not only to the epithelium covering the outside of the body, but also to the epithelium lining the oral cavity, nasal cavity, and sinuses; to the enamel of the teeth; and to the nervous system. Mesoderm gives rise to the skeletal system; muscles; blood, lymph cells, vessels; kidneys; and other internal organs. The endoderm produces the epithelial lining of the pharynx, stomach, intestines, lungs, bladder, vagina, and urethra.

These three primary embryonic layers also give rise to the structures of the face and oral cavity. The organization of the facial and oral structures will become clearer as we study the embryonic development of the face and oral cavity, and later the development of the teeth.

DEFINITION OF GROWTH AND DEVELOPMENT

Growth may be defined as an increase in the weight and spatial dimensions of an organism or organ. During growth, the organism or organ gets heavier and takes up more space. For growth the number, size, and product of cells must all increase.

Development describes an organism or organ progressing toward maturity. While the organism or organ is growing, it is maturing or becoming older. By comparing the changes of the human head (face), as depicted by the models in Figure 2-1 and the mandibular bones seen in Figure 2-2, one can understand growth and development.

THE SIZE OF A HUMAN FETUS

At the end of the third week after fertilization, the embryo is about 3 mm long. In later stages of development, the size usually is given in terms of crown-rump length. By the end of the eighth week, the crown-rump length is about 23 mm, and the embryo has acquired a form recognizable as a human being (Fig. 2-3). At the end of 3 months, the fetus[1] has a crown-rump length of about 61 mm, and at 4 months, the crown-rump length is about 116 mm.

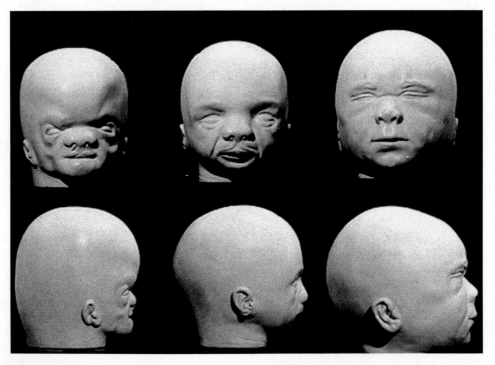

Figure 2–1. Frontal and lateral views of the human head (face). From left to right, the approximate ages represented are 10 weeks in utero, four months in utero, and birth.

---

[1] The unborn child is called an *embryo* until the end of the eighth week, after which time it is called a *fetus*.

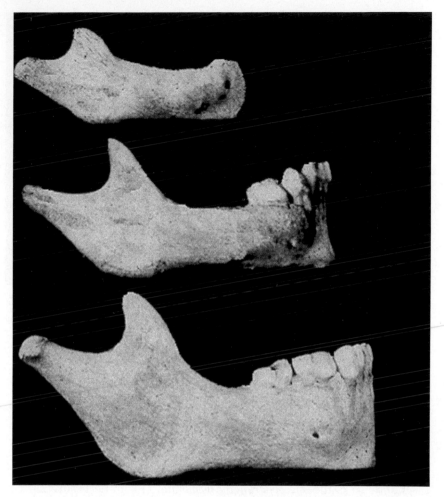

Figure 2–2. Lateral views of the mandibular bone. The term remodeling is used when referring to the growth and development of bones as organs. From top to bottom, the approximate ages of the three mandibles are one year, two years, and three years of age.

THE DEVELOPMENT OF THE FACE

The Establishment of the Primitive Mouth

Throughout embryonic development, the cephalic end of the embryo is more advanced than the caudal end. During the third week in utero, the face starts to develop as the mouth begins to form; by the end of the third week, the *stomodeum*[2] (primitive mouth) has been established. Through growth and development, the stomodeum becomes the oral and nasal cavities. (This development will be understood when studying the development of the palate.) The stomodeum forms in this manner.

---

[2] Pronounced *stō mō dē' um.*

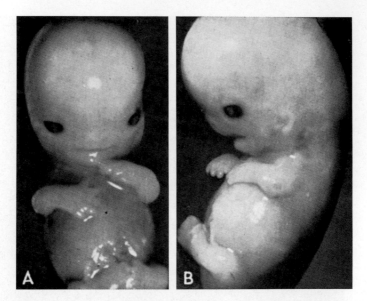

Figure 2–3. A, B. Human embryo, 25-mm long, 8 to 9 weeks old. The head is large, making up nearly half the body length. Compared with the size of the brain, the face appears small. The eyes are widespread; the ears are close to the neck; the nose is nearly flat. Notice the small size of the lower jaw. Inside the mouth of an embryo of this age, the lateral palatine processes are in a vertical position, and the tongue is tall and narrow and nearly touches the lower border of the nasal septum (see Fig. 2-12A).

On the ventral side of the cephalic end of the embryo, an invagination (an apparent pushing in) of the ectoderm occurs. This depression is the stomodeum (Figs. 2-4 and 2-5). At the deepest part of this invagination, the ectoderm is in contact with the endoderm of the *foregut* (the cephalic part of the primitive digestive tract). There is no intervening mesoderm. This combined ectoderm and endoderm is the *buccopharyngeal membrane*. (Examine Figure 2-4 carefully.) This membrane is located approximately in the region where the palatine tonsils will later appear, and it separates the primitive mouth from the foregut. The location of the buccopharyngeal membrane indicates that the stomodeum is lined with ectoderm and that the primitive digestive tract caudal to the stomodeum is lined with endoderm.

During the fourth week in utero, the buccopharyngeal membrane ruptures, thus establishing communication between the stomodeum and the primitive digestive tract. Shortly before the rupture of this membrane, about the end of the third week, a structure that is not usually thought of as being associated with the oral cavity—the *anterior lobe of the hypophysis*—begins to form. The hypophysis, or pituitary gland, is a gland of internal secretion located in the sella turcica of the sphenoid bone. It is attached to the brain, but its development starts as a small evagination of the stomodeal ectoderm (Fig. 2-4) in the roof of the primitive mouth just in front of the buccopharyngeal membrane. The pit formed by this evagination, known as *Rathke's pouch*, deepens toward the developing brain, and the cells of this pouch, derived from stomodeal ectoderm, develop into the anterior lobe of the hypophysis. The connection with the stomodeum is soon lost. The posterior lobe of the hypophysis has a different origin and is derived from the brain.

On the outside of the head, above and below the stomodeum opening, enlargements appear that will give rise to the face and to the various parts of the oral and nasal cavities.

Above the stomodeum, the recently developed forebrain causes a large bulge (Figs. 2-5 and 2-6). The ectoderm and mesenchyme that make up this bulge develop into an embryonic structure called the *frontal process*, which will give rise to the upper part of the face, the nasal septum, and the anterior part of the roof of the mouth.

Five paired branchial arches form caudal to the stomodeum, in the region of the future neck. These are ordinarily designated as branchial arches I, II, III, IV, and V (Figs. 2-7 and 2-8). Each arch is formed primarily by the migration of neural crest cells from the dorsal aspect of the developing nervous system. Neural crest cells are extremely mobile and migrate in specified "streams" beneath the head ectoderm into the developing branchial arches (Fig. 2-9). Although these cells arise from ectoderm, they become mesenchymal cells (*ectomesenchyme*) that give rise to structures such as the bones and cartilage of the head and the dentin and cementum of the teeth.

By the end of the fourth week in utero, the stomodeum has been established and the buccopharyngeal membrane has ruptured. Above the stomodeum is the frontal process, and immediately below it is the first branchial arch (Figs. 2-5 and 2-6). With the exception of the tongue, which is formed from branchial arches II,

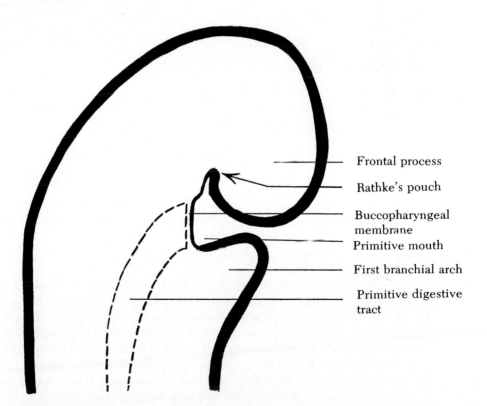

Frontal process

Rathke's pouch

Buccopharyngeal membrane

Primitive mouth

First branchial arch

Primitive digestive tract

Figure 2–4. Diagrammatic illustration of a median sagittal section through the head of a human embryo at the end of the third week in utero. Length is approximately 3 mm.

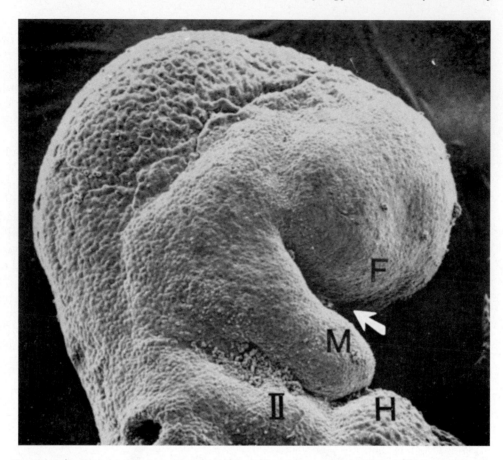

Figure 2–5. Scanning electron micrograph of a 9-day-old mouse fetus (lateral view). At this early stage, the frontal process (F) and the first branchial or mandibular arch (M) are prominent. The arrow points into the stomodeum. II, second branchial arch; H, developing heart. (Courtesy Dr. Ruth Paulson, College of Dentistry, Ohio State University.)

III, and IV, the face and all parts of the oral and nasal cavities now develop from two primary embryonic structures—the *frontal process* and the *first branchial arch*.

EARLY DEVELOPMENT OF THE FACE

The development of the face centers about the mouth. After the establishment of the stomodeum, frontal process, and branchial arches, the budding of a round process occurs on either end of the first branchial arch. These buds grow upward and medially (toward the center) at the right and left sides of the primitive mouth. They are the *maxillary processes* (Figs. 2-7, 2-8, and 2-10). After their appearance, the remaining parts of the first branchial arch are called the *mandibular processes* (Figs. 2-6, 2-7, and 2-8). Eventually the maxillary processes give rise to the upper part of the cheeks, the sides of the upper lip, and most of the palate (Fig. 2-11). The mandibular processes form the lower part of the cheeks, the lower lip, the lower jaw, and part of the tongue.

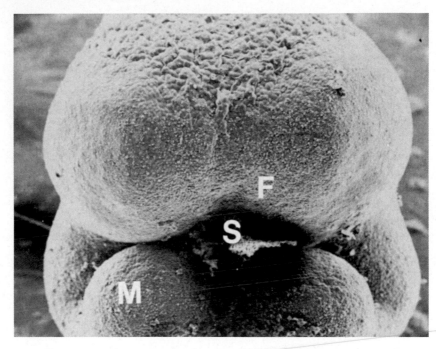

Figure 2–6. Scanning electron micrograph of a 9-day-old mouse fetus. The stomodeum (S) is bounded above by the frontal process (F) and below by the mandibular arch (M), which has not yet merged at the midline. Compare to lateral view seen in Fig. 2-5.

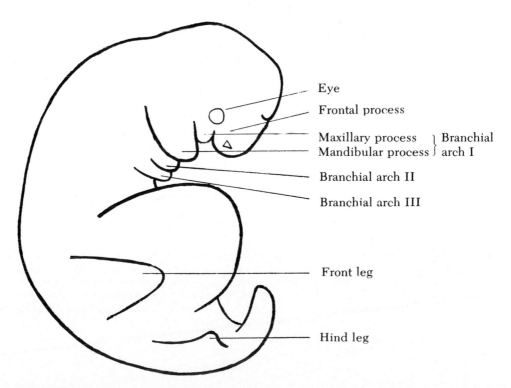

Figure 2–7. Drawing of a lateral view of a pig embryo similar to human development at about 6 weeks in utero. Branchial arches IV and V are not visible.

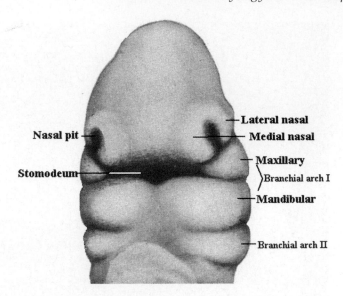

Figure 2–8. Frontal view of a pig embryo that is comparable to human development of about 6 weeks in utero.

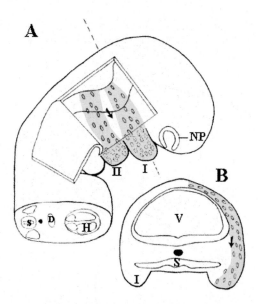

Figure 2–9. Schematic representation of the migration of neural crest cells into the branchial arches of the developing face. **A.** Lateral view of a four-week embryo with the ectoderm reflected to expose the brain stem and migrating neural crest cells. **B.** Cross section through the first branchial arch (hatched line in A) that depicts the relationship of neural crest cells to the developing nervous system and their migratory route into the mandibular arch. NP, nasal placode; S, spinal cord; D, primitive digestive tract; H, heart; V, ventricle of the brain stem, S, stomodeum.

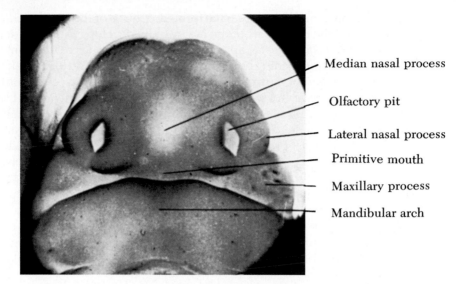

Median nasal process

Olfactory pit

Lateral nasal process

Primitive mouth

Maxillary process

Mandibular arch

Figure 2–10. Photograph of the face of a pig embryo. Length is approximately 12 mm. At this stage of development, the pig face and the human face are very much alike.

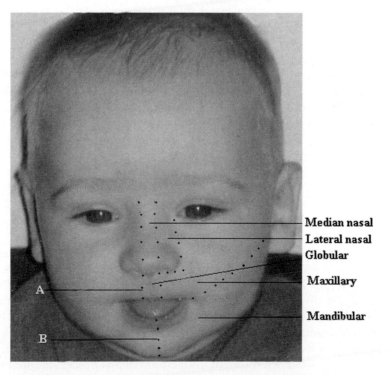

Median nasal
Lateral nasal
Globular

Maxillary

Mandibular

Figure 2–11. Photograph of a 4-month-old child's face depicting areas of the face derived from the first branchial arch and the frontal process. **A, B.** Locations at which clefts occur in the upper lip and lower jaw.

After the maxillary processes have formed, growth of the lower part of the face is retarded and the upper part of the face rapidly develops. A pair of depressions, the right and left *olfactory pits*, appears on the lower border of the frontal process. These are the future openings into the nose (Figs. 2-8 and 2-10). The olfactory pits divide the lower part of the frontal process into three parts—a center portion called the *medial nasal process* and two lateral portions called the right and left *lateral nasal processes*. The lateral nasal processes become the sides of the nose, and the median nasal process forms the center and tip of the nose (Fig. 2-11). Later, an ingrowth from the median nasal process (the center of the nose) into the stomodeum forms the nasal septum (the division between the right and left nasal chambers).

At its lower border, the median nasal process grows in length and produces a pair of bulges called the *globular process*. The globular process is not separated into two parts but remains a single median structure that grows downward to extend below the olfactory pits and lies between the right and left maxillary processes. It forms the center of the upper lip (the *philtrum*) (Fig. 2-11), and during the formation of the interior of the mouth gives rise to the anterior part of the palate, the premaxillary area (*primary palate*).

LATER DEVELOPMENT OF THE FACE

During the course of facial development, considerable *differential growth* occurs; that is, some parts grow faster than other parts. These differences in the rate of growth result in marked progressive changes in the relative size and position of the various structures. Because of the rapid growth of surrounding areas, the slower-growing median nasal process becomes relatively more narrow, and the nasal openings relatively closer together. The eyes, which appeared first on the sides of the head (Fig. 2-3), become relocated on the front of the head as a result of differential growth, while the ears change in position from the neck region to the sides of the head. For a time, the relatively slow growth of the mandibular arch results in a lag in the development of the lower part of the face. The mandible of a 2-month-old embryo (Fig. 2-3) is small in proportion to the upper part of the face.

Along with the development of the various embryonic structures, a coming together of certain of the processes occurs. The only openings that remain in the fully formed face are the openings of the mouth and nostrils; all other divisions between embryonic parts merge.

The right and left maxillary processes, which bud from the superolateral borders of the first branchial arch (Fig. 2-8), grow forward and merge with the right and left sides of the globular process. The globular process thus forms the center of the upper lip, and the maxillary processes form the sides of the upper lip (Fig. 2-11). The upper lip is completed by the end of the second month in utero.

A partial or complete failure of a maxillary process to merge with the globular process results in a condition known as *cleft lip*. Cleft lip may involve a failure of merging of the globular process with either the right or left maxillary process (unilateral) or with both the right and left maxillary processes (bilateral). A cleft lip is apparent by the end of the second month in utero, when formation of the lip is ordinarily completed.

Closure also occurs at the corners of the mouth between the maxillary and mandibular processes. This decreases the breadth of the oral opening, as mesenchyme fills in the angle formed at the junction of the mandibular processes with the right and left maxillary processes. In the adult, a line of yellow spots that frequently extends laterally along the inside of the cheek from either corner of the mouth is said to be evidence of this embryonic merger. These small yellowish elevations, called *Fordyce's spots*, are sebaceous glands. Although sebaceous glands are expected only on the outside of the body, Fordyce's spots are thought to persist in adult oral mucosa because they have become entrapped in the cheek during closure between the right and left maxillary processes with the right and left ends of the mandibular processes.

A failure of mesenchymal "flow" of the maxillary processes and the mandibular processes at the corners of the mouth leaves a cleft that results in an exceptionally large mouth opening. This anomaly is known as *macrostomia*.

Early in the life of the embryo, the deep depression originally present between the right and left sides of the mandibular processes fills at the midline. In the adult, mandibular evidence of the early existence of this depression may persist as a deep dimple in the chin. When this depression fails to fill properly during embryo development, a *median cleft* of the lower jaw (Fig. 2-11) may result. This kind of cleft is rare.

Also rare is a cleft extending from the upper lip to the eye, called an *oblique facial cleft*. Such a cleft apparently is caused when swellings of the maxillary process and the lateral nasal process fail to merge. The manner of development of this defect is at present not clear.

SUMMARY OF THE DEVELOPMENT OF THE FACE

The beginning of facial development is seen in the human embryo during the third week in utero when an invagination of the ectoderm forms the stomodeum. Above the stomodeum is the *frontal process*, and below the stomodeum is the *first branchial arch*. Buds on the superolateral border at either end of the first branchial arch form the *maxillary processes*. The first branchial arch is thus divided into two maxillary processes and two mandibular processes.

Invaginations on either side of the lower border of the frontal process, the *olfactory pits*, divide the frontal process into the *median nasal process* and the *lateral nasal processes*. The lateral nasal processes become the sides of the nose. The right and left maxillary processes grow medially from the corners of the primitive mouth and merge beneath the nose with the globular process to form the upper lip. At the corners of the primitive mouth, a filling in at the angles of the maxillary and mandibular processes reduces the size of the broad oral opening. The midline depression in the mandibular arch disappears early in development. *Differential growth* results in, among other things, a movement of the ears from the neck to the sides of the head. By the end of the second month in utero, most of these developments have taken place, but the mandible is still relatively underdeveloped.

Clefts that sometimes occur in the face as a result of faulty development include cleft lip, cleft chin, oblique facial cleft, and clefts at the corners of the mouth.

THE DEVELOPMENT OF THE ORAL CAVITY AND NASAL CAVITY

The Development of the Palate and Nasal Septum

The palate (the roof of the mouth) shows marked development near the end of the second month in utero. It arises from three sources—the right and left maxillary

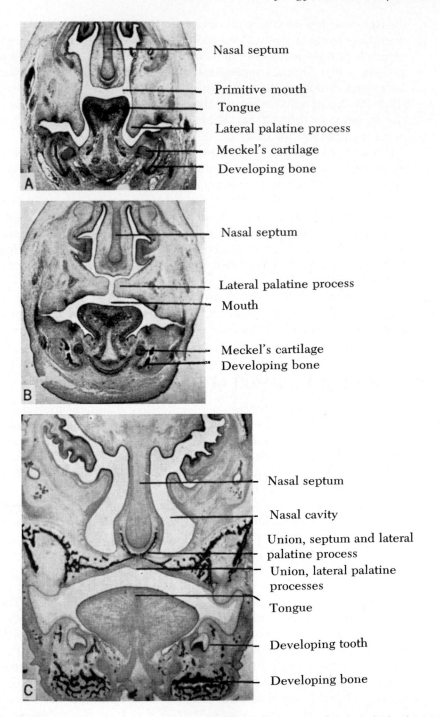

Figure 2–12. Frontal sections through the heads of 3 pigs show progressive stages in development of the palate similar to human palatal development. **A.** The vertical position of the lateral palatine processes and the position of the tongue, which nearly touches the lower border of the nasal septum, are similar to the condition in an 8-week-old human embryo (see Fig. 2-3). **B.** The lowering and broadening of the tongue, the horizontal position of the palatine processes, and their lack of union at the midline are similar to the condition in a 9-week-old human embryo. **C.** In a human fetus of 12 weeks, as in this pig fetus, the palatine processes have fused with each other and with the lower border of the nasal septum. The oral cavity and the nasal cavity are now separated by the roof of the mouth.

processes and the globular process—and forms in the following manner. Inside the stomodeum, near the end of the second month, three ingrowths appear—one from the inner surface of the right maxillary process, one from the inner surface of the left maxillary process, and one from the inner surface of the globular process (Fig. 2-12). The ingrowths into the stomodeum from the inside of the maxillary processes are called the right and left lateral palatine processes. An ingrowth from the globular process originates first as a bar of tissue inside the stomodeum between and just beneath the right and left olfactory pits. This site is approximately where the globular process arises from the median nasal process. Further ingrowth into the stomodeum develops into the *premaxillary* area of the upper jaw (primary palate). The eventual union of the two lateral palatine processes with each other (Fig. 2-13) and with the premaxillary area (Fig. 2-14) closes the Y-shaped opening in the roof of the mouth.

As these palatal structures fuse, the developing tongue becomes strangely involved. The tongue begins to develop at the end of the first month in utero. By the end of the second month, when the lateral palatine processes appear, the tongue is a comparatively large organ that extends upward into this primitive cavity until its upper surface nearly touches the lower border of the nasal septum. At first, the newly developing right and left lateral palatine processes grow vertically to the right and left of the elevated tongue (Fig. 2-12A).

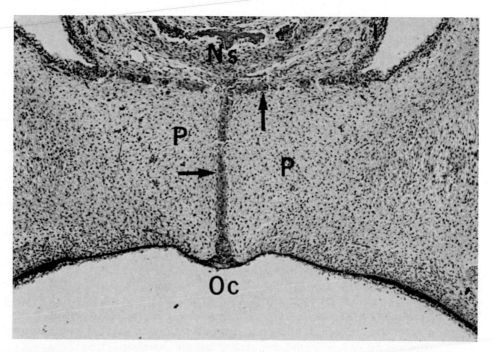

Figure 2–13. Higher magnification at the fusion sites of the horizontally positioned palatine processes (P) with each other and with the nasal septum (NS) above. The darker-staining fused epithelial cells are seen in the midline between the two palatine processes and between the palatine processes and the nasal septum. In some areas, gaps in the epithelium allow the mesenchymal cells of the structures to merge. The space on each side of the nasal septum is the nasal cavity, and the space below the palatine processes is the oral cavity. Mesenchymal cells are scattered throughout the palatine processes. The dark cells lining the oral cavity (OC) surface of the palatine processes are the oral epithelium. Refer to Fig. 2-12 for orientation.

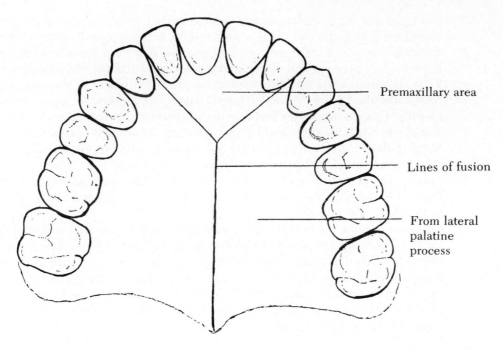

Figure 2–14. Drawing of the oral surface of a human palate. The Y-shaped lines of embryonic fusion are indicated.

The determinant of the subsequent lifting of these processes to a horizontal position (Fig. 2-12B) has been the subject of much careful study. A frequent explanation is that, as a result of enlargement of the mandible and a change in the degree of flexion of the fetus head, the tongue drops to the floor of the stomodeum. When the tongue is thus removed from the path of the growing lateral palatine processes, the processes are straightened to a horizontal position by a hinge-like movement, perhaps caused by rapid cell division at their lateral borders. Changes in position from vertical to horizontal of the lateral palatine processes occur rapidly. In the mouse embryo, this elevation takes only a few hours, and apparently it is correspondingly rapid in the human embryo.

After attaining a horizontal position early in the third month in utero, the lateral palatine processes grow medially toward each other (Fig. 2-12B), and the developing premaxillary area grows posteriorly. The palatine processes meet at the midline and fuse with each other and with the lower border of the nasal septum (Figs. 2-12C and 2-13); at their anterior borders, they meet and fuse with the posterior border of the premaxillary growth (Fig. 2-14). The structure formed is at once the roof of the oral cavity and floor of the nasal cavity, and the stomodeum has been divided into a lower chamber and an upper chamber.

The critical period for movement and complete closure of the lateral palatine processes and the premaxillary part of the palate is between 8 and 12 weeks in utero. The fusions of the roof of the mouth are normally completed by the end of 12 weeks in utero.

The palatal fusions occur as fusions of soft tissue, not of bone. Small areas of forming bone tissue are first seen in the developing palate during the eighth week in utero, when the lateral palatine processes are still in a vertical position. By the end of the third month, when the embryonic palatal structures are completely fused, bone tissue in the area is considerable, but the bones of the right and left sides of the hard palate are not together at the midline. A separation of the *bones* of the right and left sides of the roof of the mouth still exists at the end of the fourth month in utero.

As the roof of the mouth is forming, the nasal cavity becomes divided into right and left chambers by the *nasal septum*. This septum develops primarily as a growth into the stomodeum from the inside of the median nasal process. When the right and left lateral palatine processes fuse with each other in the midline of the palate, they fuse also with the inferior border of the nasal septum (Figs. 2-12C and 2-13).

Groups of epithelial cells can remain in the lines of palatal fusion to form *epithelial rests*. Epithelial rests can appear in any location at which fusion of embryonic processes occurs. These misplaced rudiments of epithelium are the origin of cysts that sometimes are found in the palatal area.

Just as a failure of one or both maxillary processes to merge with the globular process results in a cleft of the upper lip, a failure of the lateral palatine processes to fuse with each other or with the premaxillary area results in a *cleft of the palate* (Fig. 2-15). A cleft palate is apparent by the end of the third month in utero, when the palatal fusions are ordinarily completed.

Cleft palate may be slight or extensive and may involve only the uvula[3], in which case it does not affect oral function. It may involve the soft palate, a small

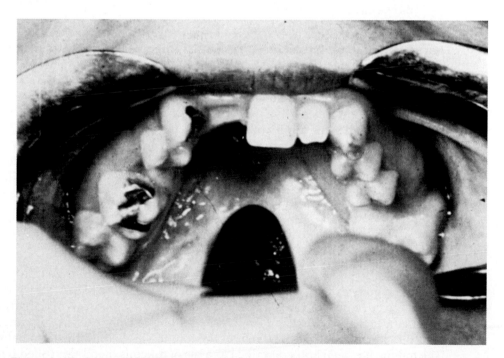

Figure 2–15. Example of an incomplete cleft of the palate. The palatine processes fused with the premaxillary area anteriorly but failed to fuse with each other posteriorly. The roof of the nasal cavity is seen in the cleft opening.

---

[3] The pendulum of soft tissue hanging down toward the base of the tongue from the center of the posterior border of the soft palate. Examine someone's mouth and see this structure.

part of the hard palate, or both the soft and hard palates. Cleft palate may also involve the alveolar ridge on one side (unilateral) or both sides (bilateral) of the midline (Fig. 2-14). Such a cleft often is located between the maxillary lateral incisor and the canine tooth, in the line of fusion between the premaxilla and the lateral palatine process; sometimes the lateral incisor is missing. In any kind of severe intraoral cleft, the maxillary teeth may be incomplete in number and often are greatly displaced. Any severe cleft of the palate also produces a crippling opening between the oral and nasal cavities, which is a serious handicap to the individual in both speaking and eating.

Cleft palate may occur with or without the presence of a cleft lip. A review of the literature on cleft lip and cleft palate in human beings has revealed substantial evidence in support of the following conclusions:

- Approximately one of every 700 newborns (5,500 newborns per year) has a cleft lip or palate.
- Cleft lip, with or without associated cleft palate, is more common in boys than in girls (65:35 ratio).
- Cleft palate is more common in girls than in boys (60:40 ratio).
- Considering all types of cleft, boys are more frequently affected than are girls (58:42 ratio).
- Clefts of the lip occur more frequently on the left side than on the right; more than 61% of unilateral clefts of the lip occur on the left side.
- Approximately 10% of individuals with facial clefts also have associated cardiovascular malformations.

A possible explanation for the greater frequency of palatal clefts in girls than in boys was deduced from a study of 46 human embryos. A time lag in the change in position of the palatal processes from vertical to horizontal apparently occurs in female embryos; consequently, female embryos may be susceptible for a longer period of time to conditions that could interfere with palatal closure.

Strong indication exists that genetic factors can determine the occurrence of cleft palate. Although some family history of clefts exists, in 20 to 30% of affected children a definite hereditary pattern has not been determined. In addition, clefts have been induced in unborn rats and mice by events that occur during the time of normal palatal closure, such as the administration of cortisone or excessive vitamin A to the pregnant females. This information obtained from animal studies cannot, of course, be applied directly to human development.

THE DEVELOPMENT OF THE TONGUE

Anatomically, the tongue has a *body* (the anterior part) and a *root* (the posterior part). The body extends from the tongue tip to the *terminal sulcus*, which is the V-shaped groove on the top surface just behind a V-shaped row of circumvallate papillae (see Fig. 10-10). (Examine someone's tongue as far back as you can see and find this row of papillae.) The root of the tongue lies behind the terminal sulcus. The tongue has been aptly described as a sac of mucous membrane filled with voluntary muscle.

When the embryo is four weeks old, the tongue begins to develop from the anterior wall of the primitive throat and protrudes upward and anteriorly. Embryologically, it develops from the region of the first four branchial arches. To picture

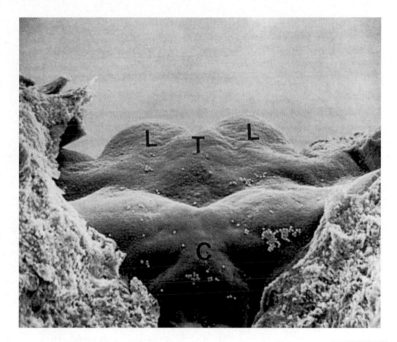

Figure 2–16. Scanning electron micrograph of a developing mouse tongue, seen from the throat region. The four lingual swellings that eventually merge to become the tongue are present. The two lateral swellings (L) and the tuberculum impar (T) are in position to form the anterior part or body of the tongue, and the single copula (C) is in place to become the posterior part or root of the tongue. (Courtesy Dr. Ruth Paulson, College of Dentistry, Ohio State University.)

its development, imagine yourself standing in the throat of a human embryo at the beginning of the second month and facing forward (Fig. 2-16). Before your eyes, near the center of the inner surface of the mandibular arch, are three recently formed lingual swellings that are aligned and will unite and become a single structure, the body or anterior part of the tongue. These three anterior swellings have specific embryonic names: The middle swelling is called tuberculum impar, and the swellings on each side are called lateral lingual swellings. Behind the three anterior swellings, in the center line between the second, third, and fourth branchial arches and involving the inner ends of these arches, is a single swelling that will become the base or root of the tongue. The embryonic name for this posterior swelling is copula. These four embryonic swellings (tuberculum impar, two lateral swellings, and copula) form the four branchial arches and unite into the single tongue, which by the end of the second month in utero has acquired a recognizable form and extends upward and forward toward the opening of the mouth (Fig. 2-17).

In the fully formed tongue, behind the *circumvallate papillae* at the tip of the V-shaped line (see Fig. 10-10), is the *foramen caecum*, a small depression that marks the point of embryonic origin of the *thyroid gland*. At about 17 days in utero, in the midline between the first and second branchial arches, the gland originates as a small proliferation of epithelium. As it develops, it descends to its final position in the neck, remaining attached to the tongue during its migration by the narrow *thyroglossal duct*. The duct eventually disappears, but the place of origin

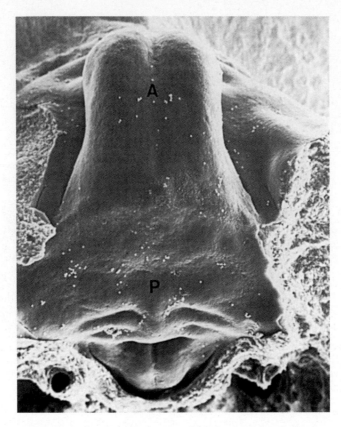

Figure 2–17. Scanning electron micrograph of a mouse tongue, seen from the throat region. The anterior (A) part of the tongue arose from the three anterior lingual swellings, and the posterior (P) part arose from the posterior single swelling seen in Fig. 2-16.

of the thyroid gland is marked on the tongue by the presence of the foramen caecum. Cell remnants of the duct can remain and give rise to thyroglossal duct cysts later in life. Typically, these are midline structures located in the region of the hyoid bone.

Bifurcation of the body of the tongue is a rare deformity and probably occurs because the lingual swellings of the first branchial arch have failed to merge. Other possible anomalies are too large a tongue (macroglossia), too small a tongue (microglossia), and absence of a tongue (aglossia). Periodically, tongue movement can be greatly restricted by the lingual frenum that connects the tongue to the floor of the mouth. This condition is referred to as ankyloglossia (tongue tied).

SUMMARY OF THE DEVELOPMENT OF THE ORAL AND NASAL CAVITIES

Table 2-1 summarizes the timing and duration of some of the major events in the formation of the human face and oral cavity. It also provides perspective on the size of the embryo at the time of these key events.

The premaxillary region of the palate develops from the globular process, a downward growth of the median nasal process, which is the center part of the orig-

TABLE 2–1. Timing of Major Events in Craniofacial Development

Developmental Structure	Duration of Presence	Size of Embryo
Stomadeum	4–9 wk	3–30 mm
Branchial arches	4–7 wk	3–17 mm
Dental lamina	4–7 wk	3–17 mm
Primary palate	4–5 wk	3–8 mm
Tongue	4–6 wk	5–12 mm
Secondary palate	7–9 wk	18–30 mm
Formation primary dentition	8–18 wk	23–135 mm
Formation secondary dentition	20 wk–5 y	160 mm

inal frontal process. The sides of the palate are formed by the lateral palatine processes. These arise from the maxillary processes, which are buds from the ends of the first branchial arch. These three structures—the premaxillary area and the right and left palatine processes—fuse in the roof of the mouth in a Y-shaped pattern (Fig. 2-14). From the part of the frontal process that forms the center of the nose (the median nasal process), the nasal septum grows back and downward, and its inferior border fuses with the right and left palatine processes as they fuse at the center of the palate (Fig. 2-13).

The tongue develops as growths from the midanterior region on the inner surface of the first four branchial arches. The body of the tongue develops from the first branchial arch; the base develops from the second, third, and fourth.

Clefts that sometimes occur inside the mouth as a result of faulty development include partial or complete clefts of the palatal structures and cleft of the tongue (Table 2-1).

SUMMARY OF THE DEVELOPMENT OF THE FACE AND ORAL CAVITY*

A summary of the derivations of the structures of the face and oral cavity is outlined in the following:

 I. Derived from the *Frontal Process* are:
  A. Median nasal process, which gives rise to:
   1. Center and tip of nose
   2. Nasal septum
   3. Globular process, which gives rise to:
    a. Philtrum of upper lip
    b. Premaxillary area of the palate
  B. Lateral nasal processes, which form:

---

* All the face and most of the structures of the oral cavity develop from two primary embryonic structures: the frontal process and the first branchial arch. The tongue alone adds to its origin the second, third, and fourth branchial arches.

        1. Sides of nose
        2. Infraorbital areas
    II. Derived from *Branchial Arch I* are:
        A. Mandibular processes, which give rise to:
            1. Lower jaw
            2. Lower parts of face
            3. Lower lip
            4. Anterior part of tongue
        B. Maxillary processes, which give rise to:
            1. Lateral palatine processes (i.e., all of palate and maxillary alveolar arch except the premaxillary area)
            2. Upper part of cheeks
            3. Sides of upper lip
    III. Derived from *Brachial Arches II, III*, and *IV*
        A. Portions of the posterior part of the tongue

SUGGESTED READINGS

Burdi AR, Silvey RG. Sexual differences in closure of the human palatal shelves. Cleft Palate J 1969;6:1–7.

Copp AJ. Prevention of neural tube defects: vitamins, enzymes and genes. Curr Opin Neurol 1998;11:97–102.

Finnell RH, et al. Neural tube and craniofacial defects with special emphasis on folate pathway genes. Crit Rev Oral Biol Med 1998;9:38–53.

Greene JC. Epidemiology of cleft lip, cleft palate. Public Health Rep. 1963;78:589.

Johnston MC, Bronsky PT. Prenatal craniofacial development: new insights on normal and abnormal mechanisms. Crit Rev Oral Biol Med 1995;6:25–79.

Moore KL, Persuad TVN. Before We Are Born: Essentials of embryology and birth defects. 5th Ed. Philadephia: W.B. Saunders, 1998.

Rothman KJ, Moore LL, Singer MR, et al. Teratogenicity of high vitamin A intake. N Engl J Med 1995;333:1369–1373.

Sadler TW. Langman's medical embryology. 7th Ed. Baltimore: Williams & Wilkins, 1995.

Slavkin HC. Incidence of cleft lips, palates rising. J Am Dent Assoc 1992;123:61–65.

Sperber GH. Craniofacial embryology. Bristol: John Wright & Sons, 1989.

3   *Tooth Development*

Before the human embryo is 3 weeks old, the stomodeum has been established. At the anterior end of the embryo, the ectoderm has invaginated to meet the endoderm, thus forming the primitive mouth and the buccopharyngeal membrane (see Fig. 2-3). This membrane is located approximately in the position that the palatine tonsils will later occupy. The primitive mouth is lined with ectoderm, beneath which is mesenchyme (ectomesenchyme, see Chapter 2). The ectoderm gives rise to the oral epithelium, and the mesenchyme becomes the underlying connective tissue.

THE BEGINNING OF TOOTH DEVELOPMENT

Odontogenesis is the name given to the origin and tissue formation of a tooth (Fig. 3-1). Not all teeth begin development at the same time. The earliest sign of tooth development in the human embryo is found in the anterior mandibular region when the embryo is five to six weeks old. Soon thereafter, evidence of tooth development appears in the anterior maxillary region, and the process progresses posteriorly in both jaws. In contrast, formation of the permanent third molars does not commence until five years of age.

A tooth arises from epithelial and connective (mesenchyme)[1] tissues of the oral cavity, both of which are derived from the ectodermal germ layer. Because the mesenchyme of the head has an ectodermal origin, it is sometimes referred to as *ectomesenchyme.* The term mesenchyme is used here with the understanding that most of the embryonic connective tissue of the head arises, not from the mesodermal germ layer as is true for the rest of the body, but from the neural crest cells as described in Chapter 2.

Development begins with the formation of the *primary dental lamina* (Figs. 3-1A, 3-2, and 3-3). The primary dental lamina is a narrow band of thickened oral epithelium (ectoderm) that extends along what will become the occlusal borders of the mandible and maxillae on a line upon which the teeth will later appear. This dental lamina grows from the surface into the underlying mesenchyme. Concurrent with the development of primary dental lamina, at 10 places in the

---

[1] Mesenchyme (pronounced *měs′ň kim*) is an embryonic connective tissue. The adjective is mesenchymal (*měs ěn′ kǐm al*).

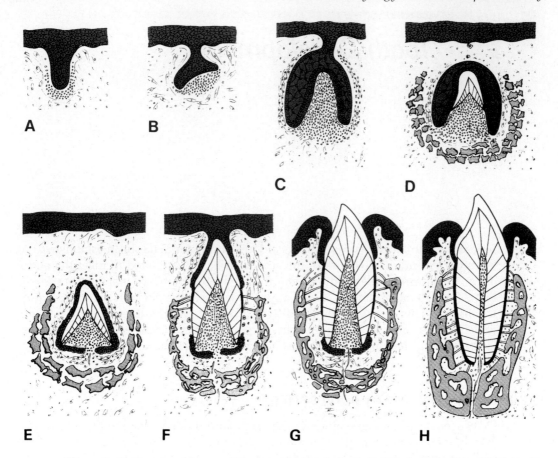

Figure 3–1. Diagram of the growth and development of a tooth. Ectodermal cells are highlighted in blue. **A.** Dental lamina stage (invagination of oral epithelium into underlying connective tissue or mesenchyme. **B.** Early enamel organ stage (budding of the epithelium of the dental lamina). **C.** Tooth germ stage (enamel organ, dental papilla, dental sac). **D.** Initiation of dentin and enamel formation within tooth germ. **E.** Reduced enamel organ and root sheath stage. **F.** Active eruption stage (breakup of root sheath and start of cementum formation). **G.** Emergence of junctional epithelium and tooth enters oral cavity. **H.** Occlusal plane stage (tooth in functional position).

Figure 3–3. Higher magnification of the primary dental lamina. The finger-like lamina (epithelium) is connected to the surrounding mesenchyme (connective tissue) by a basement membrane (arrow). Compare to Fig. 3-1A.

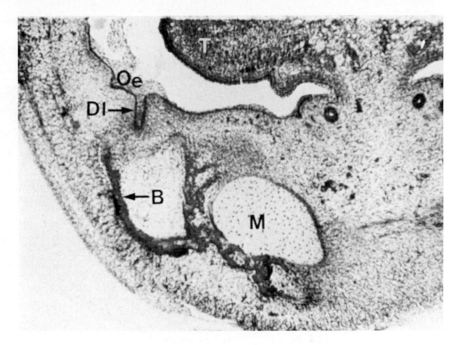

Figure 3–2. Photomicrograph of half of the lower jaw of an 8-week-old human embryo, frontal view. The primary dental lamina (DL) invaginates from the oral epithelium (OE) in the underlying mesenchyme. Here, the dental lamina appears as a finger-like process, but is actually a continuous band of epithelium that extends along the occlusal border of the jaw. B, bone of forming mandible; M, Meckel's cartilage; T, tongue. (See Fig. 3-3 for higher magnification of dental lamina.)

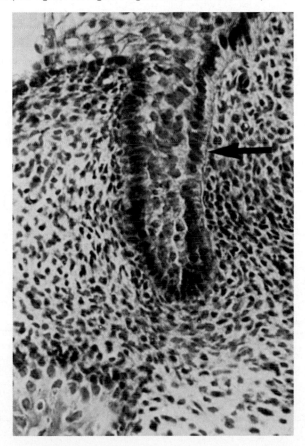

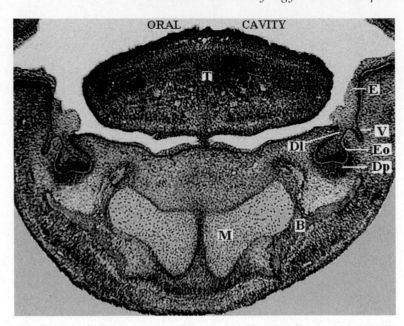

Figure 3–4. Frontal section of lower jaw in the region of the developing primary canines, 7-week human embryo. Are you able to identify the following structures on the unlabeled, left side of the jaw? DL, dental lamina; EO, early enamel organ; DP, dental papilla; E, epithelium of oral cavity; V, vestibule; B, bone of developing mandible; M, Meckel's cartilage; T, tongue.

mandibular arch and 10 places in the maxillary arch, some dental lamina cells multiply more quickly than the surrounding cells, and 10 little knobs of epithelial cells are formed on the dental lamina in each jaw. These little knobs of epithelial cells grow deeper into the underlying mesenchyme. Each of these knob-shaped structures is an early *enamel organ* (also called *dental organ*) and is the beginning of the *tooth germ* of a primary tooth (Figs. 3-1 and 3-4). Table 3-1 indicates the timing of major elements of tooth development for selected primary, permanent and suc-

TABLE 3–1. Timing of Key Events in Tooth Development

Tooth	Bud Stage of Odontogenesis	Initial Mineralization	Root Formation Complete
Primary central incisors	6 wk in utero	5 mo in utero	1.5 yr
Primary 2nd molars	8 wk in utero	6 mo in utero	3 yr
Permanent 1st molars	4 mo in utero	Birth	9–10 yr
Permanent central incisors	5 mo in utero	3–4 mo postnatal	9–10 yr
Permanent 2nd molars	10 mo postnatal	2–3 yr	14–16 yr
Permanent 3rd molars	5 yr postnatal	7–10 y	18–25 yr

cedaneous teeth. (Table 13-2 provides information on the timing of eruption for each tooth.)

The enamel organ, which is the first part of the tooth germ to form, develops from the dental lamina as a growth of oral epithelium into the underlying connective tissue (Fig. 3-4). As it enlarges, the enamel organ acquires the shape of a cap (Fig. 3-5). By the eighth week in utero, this cap formation is seen in the enamel organs of the deciduous incisor tooth germs. The connective tissue inside the cap undergoes a change and becomes the *dental papilla*. The connective tissue beneath the dental papilla becomes fibrous and encircles the papilla and part of the enamel organ, thereby forming the *dental sac (follicle)* (Figs. 3-1C, 3-6, and 3-7). The enamel organ for a time remains connected, by means of the dental lam-

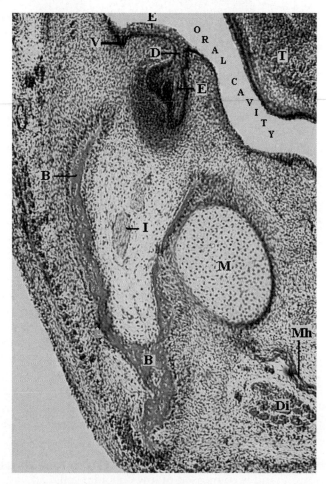

Figure 3–5. (See Color Plates) Frontal section of one side of a lower jaw in the region of the developing primary first molar, 8-week human embryo. Note the densely packed mesenchymal cells adjacent to the early epithelial enamel organ (cap); these cells will become the dental papilla and dental sac of the tooth germ. T, tongue; E, oral epithelium; V, vestibular lamina; D, dental lamina; E, early enamel organ or cap stage of tooth development; B, bone of developing mandible; I, inferior alveolar nerve; M, Meckel's cartilage; MH, mylohyoid muscle; DI, digastric muscle.

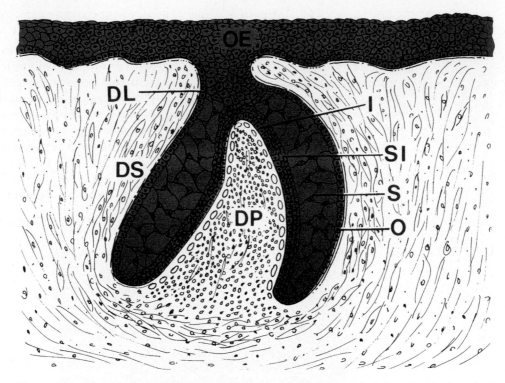

Figure 3–6. Illustration of a tooth germ. The four epithelial cell layers of the enamel organ (bell-shaped and highlighted) are indicated as I, inner; SI, stratum intermedium; S, stellate reticulum; and O, outer. The dental papilla (DP) is enclosed within four cell layers of the enamel organ and is continuous with the dental sac (DS), which surrounds the outer surface of the enamel organ. The dental lamina (DL) connects the enamel organ to the oral epithelium (OE). Compare to photomicrographs in Figs. 3-7 and 3-8.

ina, with the epithelium lining the stomodeum (Figs. 3-1C, 3-4, 3-5, and 3-6).

In summary, a tooth germ is comprised of three parts: enamel organ, dental papilla, and dental sac (follicle). The enamel organ is composed of epithelial cells that arise from the ectoderm germ layer; the dental papilla and dental sac (follicle) are connective tissues that arise from mesenchyme.

THE TOOTH GERM

As the tooth germ grows, the cap-shaped enamel organ changes form and becomes somewhat bell shaped; four layers are distinguishable (Figs. 3-6, 3-7, 3-8A, 3-8B and 3-9):

- The *outer enamel epithelium* is the outside layer of the enamel organ and is composed of low cuboidal cells.
- The *stellate reticulum* is the layer immediately inside the outer enamel epithelium and is composed of a loose network of star-shaped epithelial cells.
- The *stratum intermedium* is a layer of closely packed, flat epithelial cells inside the stellate reticulum.

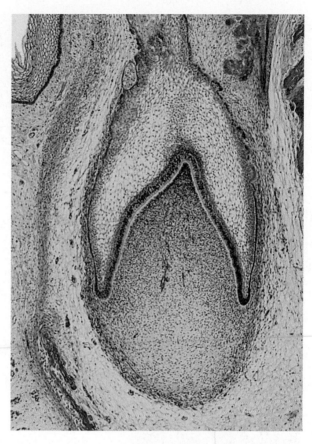

Figure 3–7. (See Color Plates) Photomicrograph of a faciolingual section of a lower incisor tooth germ. The bell-shaped enamel organ encloses the densely arranged mesenchymal cells of dental papilla. A lightly stained basement membrane lies between the enamel organ and the dental papilla and marks the future site of the dentinoenamel junction.

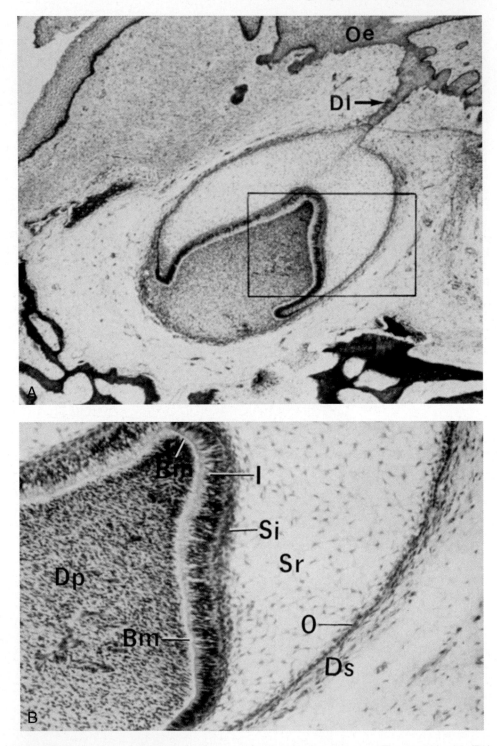

Figure 3–8. **A.** Photomicrograph of a human primary anterior tooth germ. The dental lamina (DL) still connects the epithelial cells of the enamel organ to the oral epithelium (OE). Bone of the mandible is below the tooth germ along the lower edge. **B.** Higher magnification of boxed area in Figure 3-8A. DP, dental papilla; DS, dental sac; BM, basement membrane (future site of the dentinoenamel junction); I, inner epithelial layer of enamel organ, SI, stratum intermedium; SR, stellate reticulum (widest layer); O, outer epithelial layer of enamel organ.

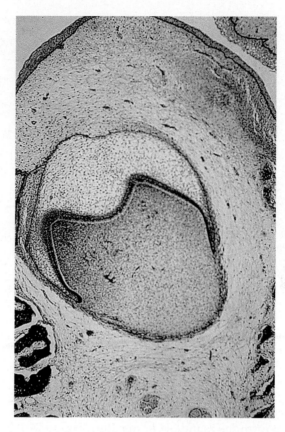

Figure 3–9. Photomicrograph of human primary molar tooth germ. The junction between the enamel organ and dental papilla is formed by a basement membrane that determines the outline and position of the dentinoenamel junction. Compare this junction outline to that of the anterior tooth germ in Fig. 3-8.

- The *inner enamel epithelium* lines the inside of the enamel organ and is composed of a single layer of cuboidal cells which are separated from the dental papilla by a *basement membrane* (Figs. 3-8B and 3-9).

Although the growing tooth germ changes form rapidly at first, by the time the four layers of the enamel organ are well-defined, the shape of the basement membrane has become fixed. The final shape of the established basement membrane marks the line that will become the dentinoenamel junction of the finished tooth (Figs. 3-8B and 3-9).

Further cell differentiation in the tooth germ occurs along either side of the basement membrane. The cuboidal cells that make up the inner enamel epithelium elongate into columnar cells called *ameloblasts*.[2] Formation of the ameloblasts is followed by a change in the peripheral cells of the dental papilla, which also take a columnar form and become *odontoblasts*. The ameloblasts and odontoblast layers are separated from each other by the basement membrane.

---

[2] Pronounced *am ĕl′ ō blāst*.

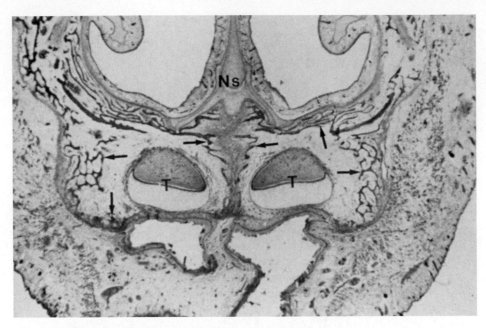

Figure 3–10. Photomicrograph showing the relation of the maxillary primary central incisor tooth germs (T) to the surrounding forming bone of the maxillae (arrows). Notice the relation of the developing teeth to the nasal cavity and the spaces on each side of the nasal septum (NS).

In embryonic development, many things occur at the same time. As the early tooth germs develop, they become surrounded by islands of bone that eventually coalesce to form the mandible or maxillae. Figure 3-10 is a mesiodistal section cut through the center of the maxillary primary incisor tooth germs. The tooth germs, which formed earlier, become enclosed in the forming bone of the maxillae. Bone of the forming mandible is clearly seen in Figures 3-11 and 3-12. Growth and de-

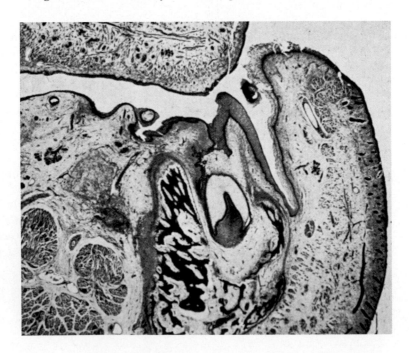

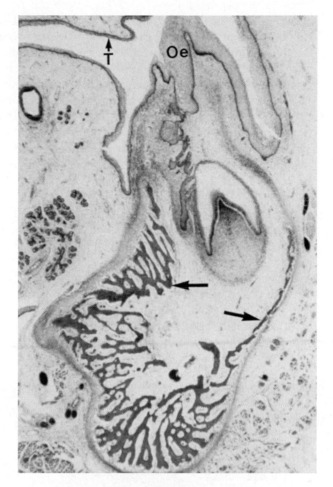

Figure 3–12. Faciolingual section through a lower primary canine tooth germ and the embryonic bone tissue of the developing mandible (arrows). Notice the spongy arrangement of the bone tissue. The developing permanent canine tooth germ is seen at the left (lingual) area of the primary tooth germ. Just below the tongue (T), a large circular opening is a cross section of the main (Wharton's) duct of the submandibular salivary gland. Refer to Fig. 3-13 for orientation and identification of the tooth germ issues. OE, oral epithelium.

velopment of the teeth and jaw bones are mutually dependent. If the rate of bone formation exceeds the rate of tooth development and eruption (tooth movements), the tooth may become impacted or firmly lodged in the jawbone. This problem, the so-called impacted wisdom tooth, frequently occurs in the third molar region. (See Chapter 13.)

By the time a primary tooth germ has reached the stage of development during which ameloblasts and odontoblasts are differentiating, other changes are taking place. Lingual to the enamel organ of the primary tooth germ, the dental lamina gives rise to the beginning of the enamel organ of the succeeding permanent tooth

---

Figure 3–11. Sagittal section of the lower jaw of the human fetus. The lower lip is on the right, and the tongue is above. A developing primary incisor tooth is becoming partially surrounded by the developing bone of the mandible.

germ (Figs. 3-13, 3-14, and 3-15). The permanent tooth germ develops slowly as the primary tooth develops and erupts into function. In addition, the dental lamina that connects both enamel organs with the oral epithelium disintegrates. The cells of the dental lamina break apart into small groups and either gradually disappear or remain as small epithelial cells. These groups of epithelial cells resemble glands histologically and are called *Serres' glands*; they are clinically significant in that they may be the source of epithelium for cysts.

The *succedaneous* enamel (dental) organs—permanent central and lateral incisors, canines, and first and second premolars—arise from the *secondary dental lamina*, which arises from the primary dental lamina (Figs. 3-14 and 3-15).

The primary dental lamina continues to invaginate from the oral epithelium posterior to the primary second molar and gives rise to the enamel organs of the permanent first, second, and third molars. The permanent molars are not succedaneous teeth (i.e., they do not replace primary teeth). The last enamel organs to appear are the third molars in about the fifth year of postnatal life. Because the third molars begin development last, they appear last in the oral cavity.

When ameloblasts and odontoblasts have differentiated along either side of the basement membrane in the tooth germ, formation of the hard

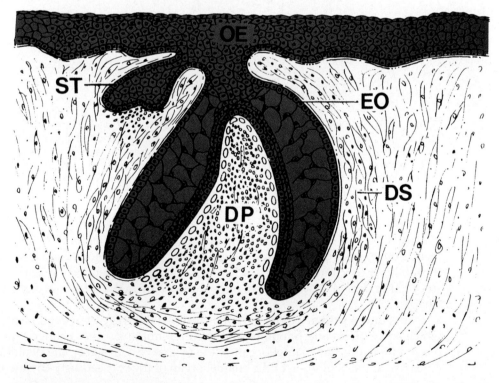

Figure 3–13. Diagram of the position of the developing succedaneous tooth (ST) lingual to the primary tooth germ. The oral lining and tooth germ epithelia are highlighted. For a comparable arrangement of the actual tissues, see Figs. 3-12 and 3-14. EO, enamel organ; DP, dental papilla; DS, dental sac; OE, oral epithelium.

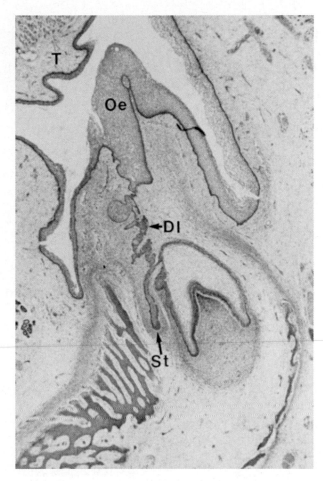

Figure 3–14. Faciolingual section of a human primary canine tooth germ and its succedaneous tooth (ST) developing lingually. Notice that the primary dental lamina (DL) is still continuous with the oral epithelium (OE); also note that the secondary dental lamina and developing enamel organ extend from the primary dental lamina. T, tongue.

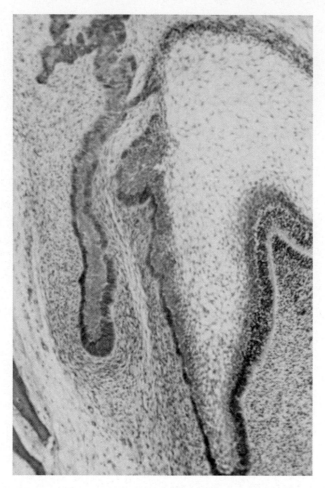

Figure 3–15. Higher magnification of the early development stage of the succedaneous tooth germ in Fig. 3-14. The four epithelial cell layers of the primary enamel organ on the right are distinct.

tooth tissues begins. The earliest formation of the hard tooth tissues in the human fetus occurs during the fifth month in the primary incisors. Dentin formation begins just before enamel formation begins.

DENTIN FORMATION

Dentin is the first mineralized tissue to appear in any developing tooth. It is composed of a fibrillar matrix that mineralizes and *odontoblastic processes* that remain unmineralized. The origin and formation of dentin is called *dentinogenesis*.

The first dentin is formed at the incisal or cusp area of a tooth; formation progresses in a rootward direction (Figs. 3-16, 3-17, and 3-18) and may be accomplished in the following manner.

The odontoblasts, which differentiated from the mesenchymal cells of the dental papilla, form a single layer of columnar cells at the line of the

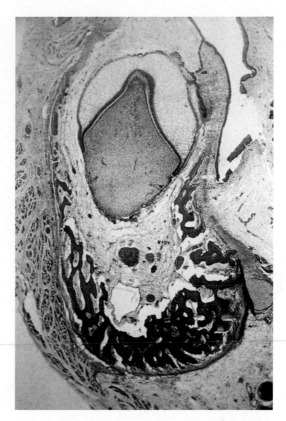

Figure 3–16. (See Color Plates) Microscopic view of the human mandibular incisor tooth germ. This tooth germ is more advanced in development than the tooth germ seen in Fig. 3-14. Dentin, the first mineralized tissue to appear in the tooth germ, is present at the coronal most part of the densely cellular dental papilla. The four cell layers of the enamel organ enclose the dentin and the cells of the dental papilla. From the lower edge of the photo to the apical part of the tooth germ is the spongy bone pattern of the mandible. The prominent round structure seen apical to the tooth germ and within the developing mandible is the inferior alveolar nerve. A higher magnification of the coronal part of the tooth germ is seen in Fig. 3-17.

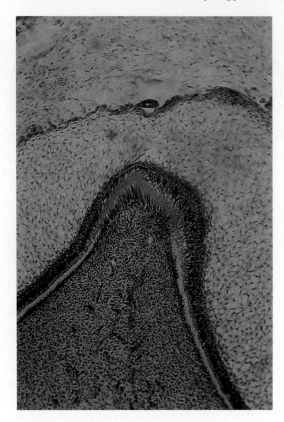

Figure 3–17. (See Color Plates) Higher magnification of the coronal part of the developing tooth seen in Fig. 3-16. The first layer of dentin is clearly seen within the topmost part of the dental papilla. The four epithelial cell layers of the enamel organ surround the dentin and the densely packed cells of the dental papilla. Refer to Fig. 3-18 for orientation and identification of tissues.

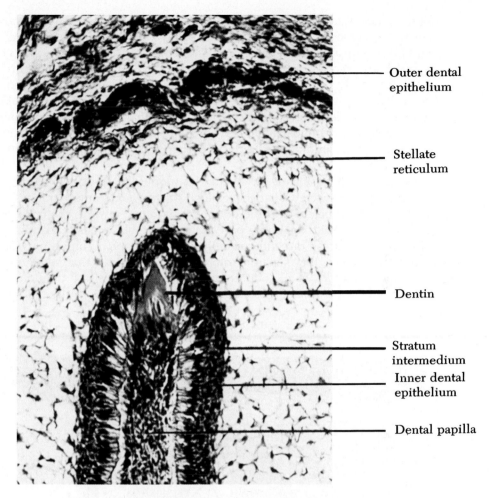

Outer dental epithelium

Stellate reticulum

Dentin

Stratum intermedium

Inner dental epithelium

Dental papilla

Figure 3–18. Enlarged histologic view of the position of the first dentin layer within the tooth germ. The four epithelial cell layers of the enamel organ are clearly visible and identified. Connective tissue of the dental sac is seen above the outer dental epithelium layer. Note that the stellate reticulum layer remains conspicuously wide compared with the outer layers of the enamel organ.

dentinoenamel junction (Figs. 3-19 and 3-20). They begin moving inward, back toward the center of the pulp. The cells behave as though several spots of their cytoplasm were attached to the basement membrane, thus causing the cytoplasm to stretch out into several narrow extensions (Fig. 3-21). As the pulpward migration of the body of the odontoblasts progresses, the cytoplasmic extensions of each cell join to make a single dentinal process. The part of the odontoblasts that contains the nucleus comes to rest somewhat pulpal to the basement membrane (soon to be the dentinoenamel junction), but the cells remain connected with their point of origin by the cytoplasmic extensions, which are branched at their peripheral ends.

When the odontoblasts differentiated along the periphery of the dental papilla, heavy corkscrew-shaped collagen fibers were formed among them. As dentin formation begins and the odontoblasts move inward, the collagen fibers remain in place. With the bulky part of the odontoblast cells out of the way, the collagen fibers spread out and resemble a piece of rope becoming unwound and frayed. In this way, they separate into tiny collagen fibrils that lie among the cytoplasmic extensions of the odontoblasts. These fibrils of the dentin matrix are surrounded by the *ground substance of the dentin matrix.* Both the collagen fibers

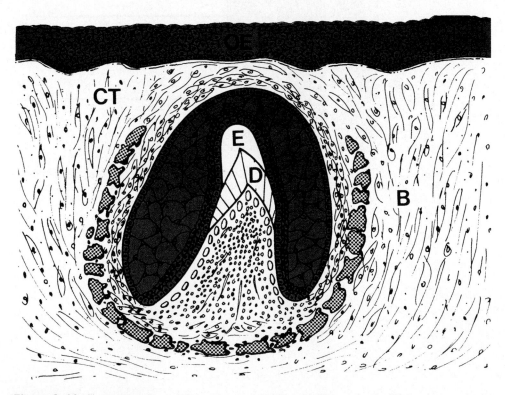

Figure 3–19. Illustration of an advanced tooth germ. Enamel (E) and dentin (D) are present in the coronal most area. Ameloblasts are present around the enamel, whereas cervically the inner epithelial cells have not yet differentiated into ameloblasts. The dental sac surrounds the enamel organ and is continuous with the dental papilla. Developing bone (B) of the jaw is present, and the developing tooth is separated from the epithelium (OE) by connective tissue (CT). Compare to photomicrograph in Fig. 3-20.

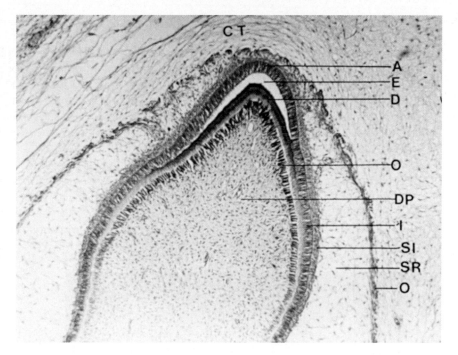

Figure 3–20. Photomicrograph of an advanced tooth germ. The coronal most part of the tooth germ is more differentiated that the apical part. Coronally, ameloblasts (A) are seen, and the enamel (E) matrix has formed, along with dentin (D) and odontoblasts (O), in the dental papilla (DP). Apically, the four epithelial cell layers are clearly seen: inner (I), stratum intermedium (SI), stellate reticulum (SR), outer (O). Note the surrounding connective tissue (CT) and the absence of the dental lamina.

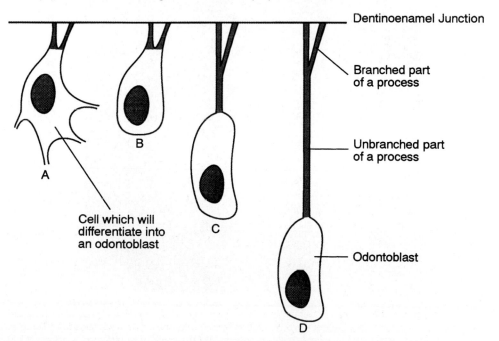

Figure 3–21. Schematic diagram of the possible manner of formation of an odontoblastic process. **A.** A pulp cell, which will differentiate into a columnar odontoblast. **B.** The odontoblast has moved away from the dentinoenamel junction, but part of its cytoplasm remains stretched behind in two places. **C.** The odontoblast has moved farther inward, and its cytoplasmic processes have united. **D.** The odontoblast has moved still farther inward, and a long cell process has been formed.

and the ground substance (*organic matrix*) are produced by the odontoblasts. The cytoplasmic extensions of the odontoblasts are the odontoblastic processes.

The dentin matrix mineralizes progressively as it is produced. The innermost layer of the dentin matrix, located next to the pulp, is the most recently formed, and in developing teeth this layer is not mineralized until a successive layer has been formed. This newest, nonmineralized dentin is called *predentin* or *dentinoid* (Figs. 3-22 and 3-23).

Dentin may be produced along the pulpal wall in a tooth of any age as long as the pulp is intact. Dentin formed in older teeth in response to attrition or caries is called *reparative dentin*. The tubules in reparative dentin are fewer and less regular in arrangement than are those of earlier dentin because, as a result of changes in the pulps of older teeth, fewer odontoblasts, and thus fewer odontoblastic processes, exist.

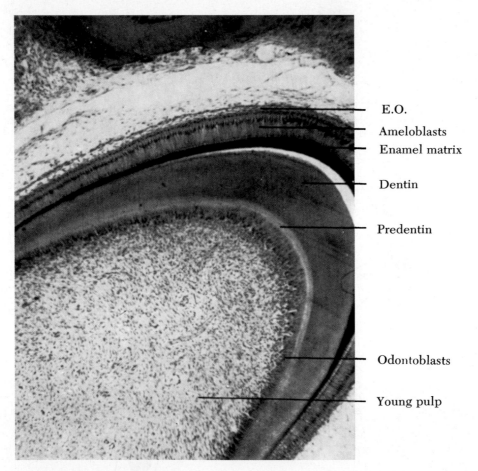

Figure 3–22. Photomicrograph of a developing mandibular tooth (cusp tip) of a kitten. Odontoblasts lie around the periphery of the pulp. Outside of the odontoblasts is light-stained predentin then darker-stained dentin. The space between the dentin and the black enamel matrix is artifact. Outside of the enamel matrix are the tall, columnar ameloblasts with their nuclei located at their outer ends. Outside of the ameloblasts the outer three layers of the enamel organ (EO)—stratum intermedium, stellate reticulum, outer enamel epithelium—have been reduced to a few layers of flat cells. When the enamel matrix is completely formed, the ameloblasts become similarly flattened. The four indistinguishable layers are then collectively the reduced enamel epithelium, as in Fig. 3-25.

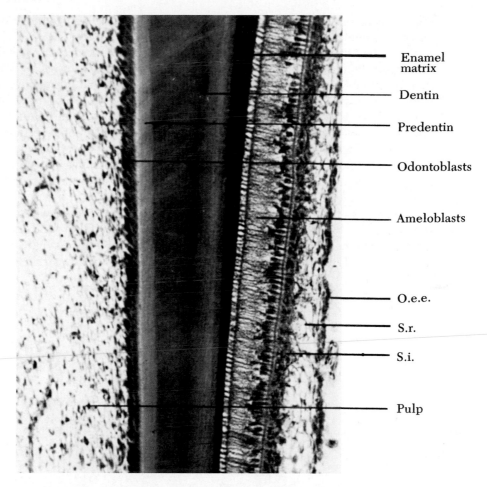

Enamel matrix

Dentin

Predentin

Odontoblasts

Ameloblasts

O.e.e.

S.r.

S.i.

Pulp

Figure 3–23. Higher magnification of the cervical ameloblasts. This tooth is at roughly the same stage of development as the tooth in Fig. 3-25. Note the regular arrangement of the tall columnar ameloblasts. Compare the ameloblasts to the smaller cell bodies of the odontoblasts. These cells move in opposite directions during formation of the matrix. OEE, outer enamel epithelial layer; SI, stratum intermedium layer; SR, stellate reticulum layer.

When dentin formation begins, the forming organ is called the dental papilla. After some amount of dentin has been produced, the dental papilla is referred to as *dental pulp*.

ENAMEL FORMATION

Tooth enamel is a product of the enamel organ. The ameloblasts, which earlier in development were the inner enamel epithelial cells of the enamel organ, produce an organic enamel matrix in which mineral salts later crystallize out of solution and form the hard enamel. The origin and formation of enamel is called *amelogenesis*.

Enamel matrix formation begins soon after the beginning of dentin formation, at the dentin surface (or incisal edge) of the cusps, and closely follows the progress of dentin formation. As the odontoblasts of the pulp move inward and leave behind a cell process and dentin matrix, the opposing ameloblasts move outward, leaving enamel matrix in their wake (Figs. 3-22, 3-23, 3-24 and 3-25).

Enamel matrix is laid down in the form of enamel rods and inter-rod substance. The organic matrix is a product of ameloblast. As ameloblasts move away from the dentinoenamel junction, they deposit drops of material that remain in a line and resemble a string of flattened beads in close union (see Fig. 4-6). This drop formation is believed to produce the apparent segments, or units, of the enamel rods that are seen as cross-striations when mature teeth are ground into thin sections and examined under a high power microscope. The inter-rod substance between the enamel rods is a product of the intercellular substance that lies between and is secreted by the ameloblasts. Current thinking is that the organic matrix of one enamel rod may be formed by more than one ameloblast.

After the matrix has formed, enamel formation is completed when submicroscopic crystals or inorganic substances develop among and around the fibrils of the matrix of the rods and inter-rod substance. These crystals have distinct orientations. Crystals in the center of the rods lie with their long axes parallel to the long

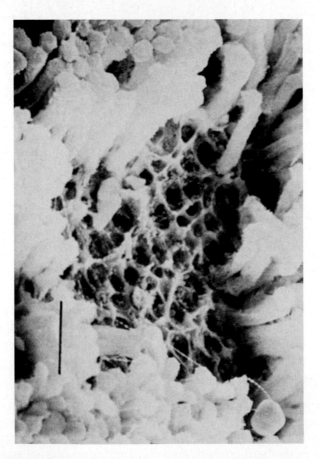

Figure 3–24. Scanning electron micrograph of ameloblasts. Here, the ameloblasts are seen as white columnar cells, which move towards the viewer as they form the underlying enamel matrix. The honeycomb-appearing matrix is seen in the center, where the ameloblasts were lost during specimen processing. The marker represents 20 mm. (Courtesy Dr. Dennis Foreman, College of Dentistry, Ohio State University.)

Oral epithelium

Reduced enamel
epithelium

Enamel matrix

Dentin

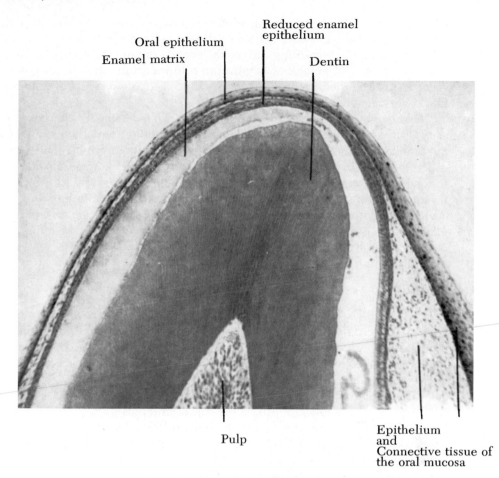

Pulp

Epithelium
and
Connective tissue of
the oral mucosa

Figure 3–25. Anterior tooth of a fetal pig. With slightly more occlusal movement, the tooth tip will break through into the oral cavity. Around the edge of the breakthrough, the oral epithelium and reduced enamel epithelium will become united and protectively seal in the connective tissue. After the emergence of the tooth, the reduced enamel epithelium will be referred to as attachment epithelium. The enamel matrix on the right side of the picture was washed away in section preparation. At this stage, calcification of enamel is well advanced. Notice the resemblance of this tooth to the kitten tooth in Fig. 3-22.

axes of the rods; crystals between the rods—in the inter-rod substance—lie at an angle to the long axes of the rods. Tooth enamel, which is approximately 96% mineral substance, is the hardest of all body tissues.

After the ameloblasts have completed the production of the enamel matrix, some histologists believe that they produce a smooth coating over its surface. This coating, called the *primary enamel cuticle*, mineralizes and covers the entire surface of the tooth crown. The primary enamel cuticle is not visible in ground sections of tooth enamel and thus is not shown in any of the illustrations in this book.

The destiny of the enamel organ of the tooth germ is important. As the enamel matrix is being produced and the ameloblasts are moving from the dentinoenamel junction, the stellate reticulum of the enamel organ narrows and becomes indiscernible. The enamel organ is reduced to a layer of ameloblasts plus a few layers of squamous epithelial cells, which are the remains of the rest of the enamel organ

(Figs. 3-1E and 3-23). When the ameloblasts have completed formation of the matrix of the enamel rods, they become flattened epithelial cells and blend indistinguishably with the remaining cells of the enamel organ. The enamel organ, originally composed of ameloblasts, stratum intermedium, stellate reticulum, and outer enamel epithelium, has thus been reduced to a few layers of flattened cells that cover the newly formed tooth crown.

These combined layers of cells are called the *reduced enamel epithelium,* or *reduced dental epithelium* (Fig. 3-25). The reduced enamel epithelium now produces a nonmineralized enamel cuticle over the surface of the tooth crown. This product is called the *secondary enamel cuticle,* or *dental cuticle,* which surrounds and protects the enamel of the tooth until the enamel emerges into the oral cavity (Fig. 3-25). After the tooth tip emerges, the part of the reduced enamel epithelium that remains surrounding the crown is referred to as the *junctional epithelium,* or *attachment epithelium.* The junctional epithelium of a newly erupted tooth is the remnant of the original enamel organ of the tooth germ (see Fig. 3-1).

ENAMEL SPINDLES

Enamel spindles (Figs. 4-20 and 4-21) originate in the early tooth germ before the cells that derive from ectoderm and mesenchyme have differentiated into ameloblasts and odontoblasts. Some of the cells that are to become odontoblasts have thin projections of cytoplasm crossing the line that will become the dentinoenamel junction and lying among the cells that will become ameloblasts. After cell differentiation, the odontoblasts move inward as dentin matrix is formed. As they move their cytoplasmic projections, the odontoblasts stretch out into what are called odontoblastic processes, but the ends of the processes remain among the ameloblasts. When enamel matrix forms and mineralizes, the ends of the odontoblastic processes are the so-called *spindles.* In older teeth, the spindle most likely becomes a space that once held odontoblast cytoplasm.

ROOT FORMATION

Formation of dentin and enamel begins in the incisal or cuspal areas of the tooth and progresses cervically. Enamel formation stops at the termination of the enamel organ, which is the cervical border of the tooth crown. Dentin formation continues beyond this point, and the dentin of the root is formed (Fig. 3-1F, G). As the root dentin begins to form, the already formed tooth crown moves occlusally, although the tooth does not emerge into the oral cavity until a considerable portion of the root has been produced. If the tooth has a single root, the dentin wall encloses a single pulp canal. If the tooth is multirooted, the division of the pulp cavity into two pulp canals, each surrounded by a wall of dentin, is apparent soon after the completion of the crown. Figure 3-26 is a photograph of a mandibular third molar from which the buccal wall has been removed. The crown of this tooth is complete. Dentin has formed beyond the cervical border of the enamel, and a short root trunk is present. The center of the lower edge of this young tooth pulp contains evidence of its division into two branches, one for the mesial root and one for the distal root. Figure 3-27 is a similar tooth, the roots of which are slightly more advanced in development. Here the root bifurcation is obvious. Drying of the specimen during preparation causes the tooth pulp in

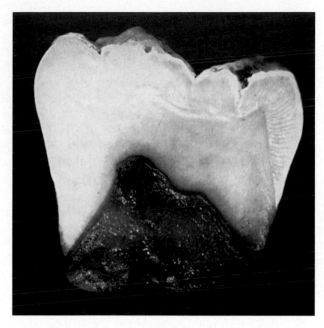

Figure 3–26. Mandibular left third molar, buccal side removed. The crown of this tooth is completed, and the root has started to form. The lower border of the pulp chamber shows the beginning of a division into two root canals.

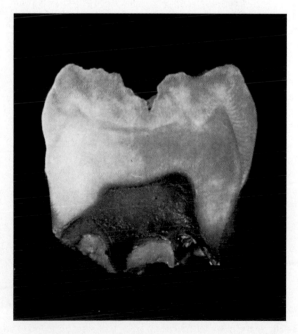

Figure 3–27. Mandibular right third molar, buccal side removed. The crown is completed, and the beginning development of two roots is clear.

each root to shrink at its lower border, thereby erroneously revealing four developing roots at first glance.

Figure 3-28 is a photograph of a mandibular third molar, the roots of which have attained approximately three fourths of their final length. The root canals are broad, and their apical openings are large.

Figure 3-29 is a photograph of the buccal surface of a mandibular third molar, the roots of which are approximately about two thirds of their final length. The apical openings are large. In the process of studying extracted teeth, students often mistake the short, square shape of such roots as an indication of partial root resorption. A permanent tooth with the apical third of its roots resorbed would have small root canals (because it probably would be an older tooth), and the root ends most likely would not have this square shape.

Figure 3-30 is a tooth similar to the tooth shown in Figure 3-29. The perspective of this picture looks up into the open ends of the root canals. Notice the large size of the root canals and the thinness of the dentin wall.

Root length is not complete until one to four years after the tooth emerges into the oral cavity. A newly emerged tooth has a short root and a large apical opening. As teeth become older, the root length is completed and additional dentin continues to form on the pulpal surface of the existing dentin until the root canal becomes narrow and the apical opening becomes small. The stage of development of the root (i.e., the size of the root canal and apical foramen) is important to the dentist if an accident or dental caries makes endodontic treatment necessary.

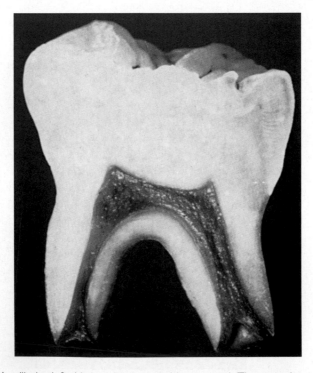

Figure 3–28. Mandibular left third molar, buccal side removed. The roots have attained approximately three fourths of their length. The root canals are broad, and the opening at the ends of the incompletely formed roots are large.

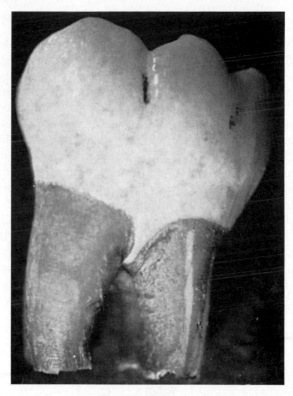

Figure 3–29. Buccal surface of a left mandibular third molar. The roots have attained approximately two thirds of their length. The openings at the ends of the incompletely formed roots are large. In this tooth, the enamel extends between the roots and meets the enamel on the lingual surface of the tooth.

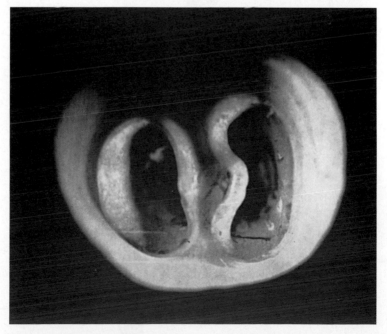

Figure 3–30. A mandibular second molar. This picture was taken looking into the large openings at the ends of the incompletely formed roots.

FORMATION OF PERIODONTAL LIGAMENT AND CEMENTUM

As dentin is forming apical to the cervical line of the enamel, the circularly arranged fibers of the dental sac become the periodontal ligament around the tooth root. The periodontal ligament produces the cementum that covers the root dentin and the lamina dura of the tooth socket. As the cementum and lamina dura are being produced about the forming root, fibers of the periodontal ligament become entrapped in their substance. The attachment of the periodontal ligament fibers in the lamina dura and cementum holds the tooth securely in the socket (Fig. 3-1). As the tooth erupts, the periodontal ligament fibers are reoriented.

As the tooth crown moves occlusally, it carries the reduced enamel epithelium that covers it. At the cervical border of the reduced enamel epithelium, some of its cells seem to pull off in strands that remain stretched like a network in the periodontal ligament around the forming root. This network is called *Hertwig's epithelial root sheath.* The root sheath determines the outline of the root dentin before cementum formation begins and determines the number of roots a tooth will have. The cells of Hertwig's epithelial root sheath must break up and pull away from the root dentin surface before the cementoblasts can move to the surface and produce the cementum matrix (Figs. 3-1, 3-31, 3-32, and 3-33). Later, when the tooth is fully

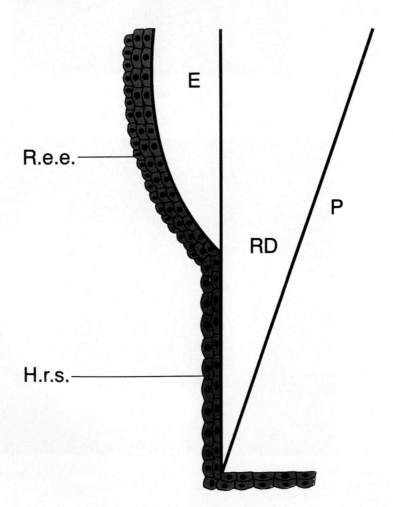

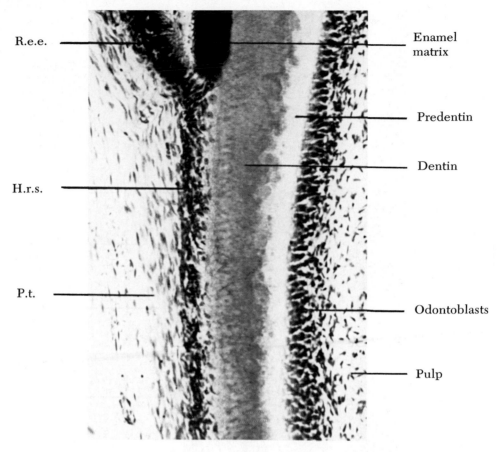

R.e.e.

H.r.s.

P.t.

Enamel
matrix

Predentin

Dentin

Odontoblasts

Pulp

Figure 3–32. Photomicrograph of the cervical region of a developing kitten tooth. Hertwig's epithelial root sheath (HRS) is still intact along the root dentin and still continuous with the reduced enamel (dental) epithelium (REE) over the crown. Cementum is not present at this stage of development. Hertwig's sheath must break up and pull away from the root dentin surface before the cementoblasts can move to the surface and produce the cementum matrix. PT, periodontal tissue. Compare to Fig. 3-31.

Figure 3–31. Diagram of the relationship of the remaining epithelial cells of an enamel organ to a tooth surface. Over the enamel (E), cells are arranged as the reduced enamel epithelial layer (REE), and over the root dentin (RD), the cells are arranged as the two-layered Hertwig's epithelial root sheath (HRS). P, pulp. See Figs. 3-32 and 3-33 for histologic views of tissues.

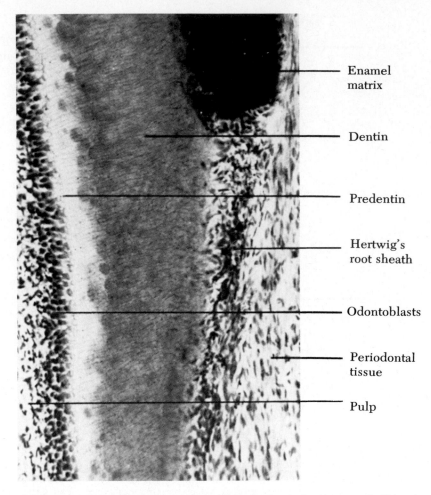

Enamel
matrix

Dentin

Predentin

Hertwig's
root sheath

Odontoblasts

Periodontal
tissue

Pulp

Figure 3–33. Photomicrograph of the cervical region of a developing kitten tooth. This microscopic view is similar to that seen in Fig. 3-31, but in a more advanced stage. Hertwig's epithelial root sheath cells are separated and less concentrated, especially in the most cervical root area just apical to the enamel matrix. Here, cementoblasts from the dental sac have moved to the root dentin surface and have begun to form cementum.

formed and in function, a few fragments of Hertwig's epithelial sheath may still be found upon microscopic examination of the periodontal ligament. These small groups of cells are called the epithelial *rests of Malassez*. (See Chapter 8.)

ANOMALIES

Development of the teeth may vary in several ways from the standard. When fewer than the normal number of tooth germs develop, an individual may have too few teeth (*hypodontia*) or no teeth (*anodontia*). When more than the usual number of tooth germs develop, the individual may have too many teeth, which are called *supernumerary teeth* (super = additional; numerary = number) (Fig. 3-34). Sometimes certain teeth have a peculiar shape: the maxillary lateral incisor may be peg-shaped, or the maxillary central incisor may be screwdriver-shaped, having a

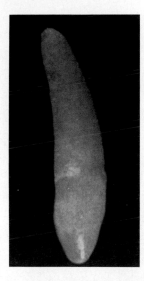

Figure 3–34. A supernumerary tooth (history unknown). This kind of tooth is usually found in the maxilla, lingual to other teeth.

mesiodistal dimension that is smaller in the incisal third than in the cervical portion.

Again, development of the hard tooth tissues may be faulty. Enamel development may be so imperfect that the enamel is lost from the surface of the tooth soon after eruption; this condition is hereditary. A more frequent condition is localized enamel hypoplasia (hypo = under; plasia = formation), which results from a systemic disturbance during tooth crown formation. This condition is often seen in the form of a pitted line across the facial surfaces of the permanent incisors, the tips of the canines, and the cusps of the first molars in the same mouth. It affects the areas of the teeth that were in the process of formation during the systemic hypoplasia.

Still another abnormality results from interference with the calcification of the enamel matrix, which produces hypomineralized areas in the enamel. This condition is seen in individuals who have lived during the first 8 years of their lives in regions where the drinking water contained over 2 parts per million (ppm) of fluoride. Fluoride in the drinking water causes enamel hypomineralization only when it is consumed during the period of tooth formation; such hypomineralization is clinically visible only when the fluoride exists in amounts in excess of approximately 2 ppm. When they are exposed to the oral cavity, the hypomineralized areas of enamel become stained with brown unsightly. This condition is called *mottled enamel* or *dental fluorosis* (Fig. 3-35).

Another variation in enamel formation found in molars, chiefly mandibular molars, is an extension of the enamel at its cervical border between the roots of the teeth (Fig. 3-36). This pattern of enamel distribution has been reported in 90% of the mandibular first molars in persons of Mongoloid racial stock but is unusual in teeth of persons of Caucasoid racial stock.

An interesting anomaly sometimes seen during examination of a collection of extracted teeth is the *enamel pearl*. This spot of enamel, usually in the shape of a half-sphere, is found on the roots of teeth, most frequently on the distal surface of

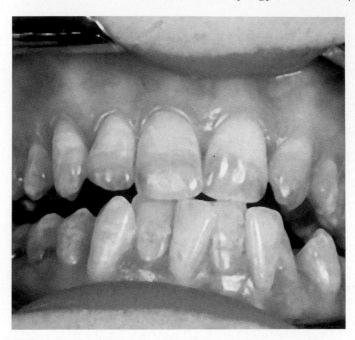

Figure 3–35. (See Color Plates) Clinical view of mottled enamel or dental fluorosis. Note that the teeth appear normal except for the brown-stained, hypomineralized areas caused by excessive exposure to fluoride during the period of enamel formation.

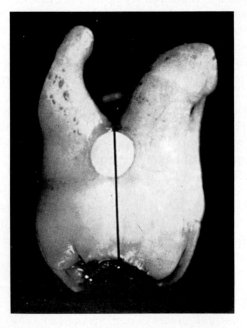

Figure 3–36. Distal surface of a maxillary right third molar. An enamel pearl is seen on the root trunk. The tooth was ground to a thin section along the vertical line. See also Fig. 3-38.

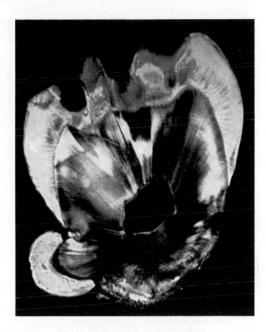

Figure 3–37. A ground section of the tooth shown in Fig. 3-36. The enamel pearl is in the upper right. The roots are not present here because the section was made at the root furcation. Notice that, in addition to a formation of enamel in this unusual location, a variation in the dentin formation has resulted in a protrusion of dentin beneath the enamel pearl.

third molars (Figs. 3-36, 3-37, and 3-38), and less frequently on the buccal surface of a molar at the root of furcation. The formation of enamel pearls is ordinarily said to result when a small group of cells of Hertwig's epithelial root sheath adhere to the surface of the newly formed root dentin instead of separating from the dentin and moving out into the periodontal ligament. Like the cells of the inner enamel epithelium in the crown area, these epithelial cells that adhere to the root dentin differentiate into ameloblasts, and a drop of enamel (enamel pearl) is then produced on the root.

Because the dentin beneath the enamel pearl in many, if not all, cases protrudes into the pearl, the production of an enamel pearl is more than the cells of Hertwig's sheath merely adhering to the root dentin. That is, the external dentin surface is not flat, as on the rest of the root; a protrusion of dentin is covered by the enamel pearl (Figs. 3-39 and 3-40B). In some teeth, the configuration of the pulp canal is also altered. In the cross section of the tooth shown in Figure 3-39, an extrusion of the wall of the pulp canal lies beneath the enamel pearl.

Sometimes a tooth root reveals a projection larger than an enamel pearl and is comprised of an enamel-covered crown and a short cementum-covered root (Fig. 3-40A). This projection, an attached supernumerary tooth, results from anomalous formation of the tooth germ at an early stage of development. In such a specimen, the pulp cavities of the large tooth and supernumerary tooth are usually united (Fig. 3-40B). (Compare the pulp cavities of the specimens in Figs. 3-39 and 3-40B.)

Figure 3-41 is a supernumerary tooth between or among the roots of a mandibular third molar. This mandibular molar has a third root beneath the distolingual

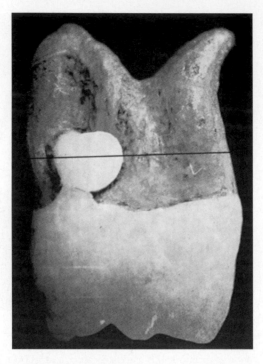

Figure 3–38. A maxillary right third molar with a large enamel pearl on the distal surface of the lingual root. The tooth was ground to a thin section along the horizontal line. (See also Fig. 3-41.)

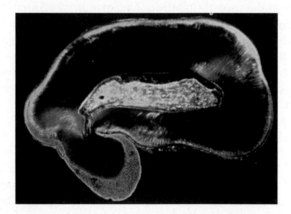

Figure 3–39. A ground section of the tooth shown in Fig. 3-38. The enamel pearl is in the lower left. In this tooth, not only is a protrusion of the dentin beneath the enamel pearl, but also an extrusion of the pulp cavity is in the location of the pearl.

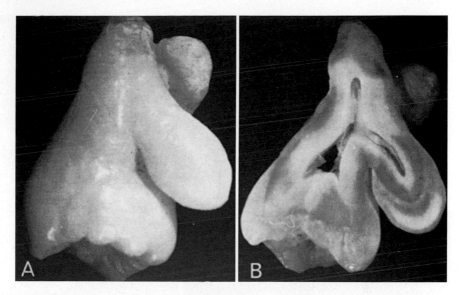

Figure 3–40. A. Buccal aspect of a left maxillary third molar with a supernumerary tooth growing from its distal side. **B.** When the buccal surface was ground away, the pulp cavities of the third molar and the supernumerary tooth were found to be joined.

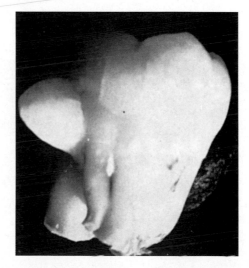

Figure 3–41. Lingual aspect of a left mandibular third molar with a supernumerary tooth between its roots. The crown of the supernumerary tooth is pointed distolingually. Notice the small extra root on the lingual side of the molar.

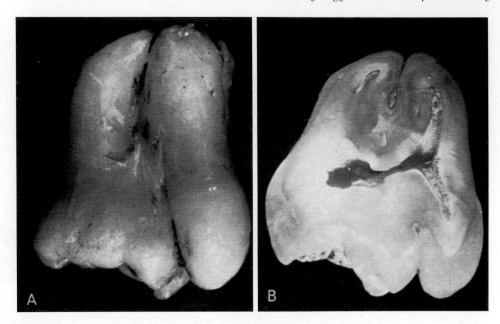

Figure 3–42. A. Distal aspect of the right maxillary third molar. A supernumerary tooth is attached to the buccal surface of the distobuccal cusp. **B.** The distal side of the tooth was ground off and exposed the united pulp cavities.

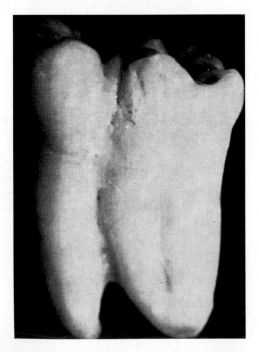

Figure 3–43. Careful study of this anomaly failed to reveal its probable location in the mouth other than that it clearly came from the mandibular molar area. The buccal and lingual aspects could not be identified with any confidence.

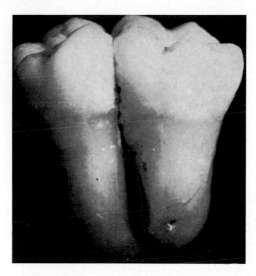

Figure 3–44. The lingual surface of fused mandibular molars.

cusp. When one side of the specimen was ground away, the pulp cavities of the molar and supernumerary tooth were found to be united.

Figure 3-42A is a right maxillary third molar with a supernumerary tooth attached to the buccal surface of the distobuccal cusp and root. When the distal side of the tooth was removed, the pulp cavities were seen to be united (Fig. 3-42B).

Figure 3-43 is a picture of fused mandibular molars, the pulp cavities of which form a common chamber.

Although the specimen of fused mandibular molars seen in Figure 3-44 contain only two roots externally and two root canals internally, two distinct crowns were fused, each with two buccal and two lingual cusps. The pulp chambers in the crowns were united.

The shape of these kinds of anomalies is established during the early stages of the formation of the enamel organ. Before any matrix of hard tissue is produced in a developing tooth, the enamel organ takes a shape such that the cells of the inner enamel epithelium, which become ameloblasts, have the configuration of the future dentinoenamel junction. The basement membrane, located between the ameloblasts and the peripheral cells of the dental papilla, is the location of the future dentinoenamel junction. In the developing tooth, many of these anomalies are visible upon examination of microscopic sections.

SUGGESTED READINGS

Ten Cate AR. Oral histology: development, structure, and function. 5th Ed. St. Louis: Mosby; 1998.

Thesleff I. Two genes for missing teeth. Nat Genet 1996;13:379–380.

Weiss KM, Stock DW, Zhao Z. Dynamic interactions and evolutionary genetics of dental patterning. Crit Rev Oral Biol Med 1998;9:369–398.

Tooth Development Group of the Developmental Biology Programme, Institute of Biotechnology, University of Helsinki. Gene expression in tooth. Available at: http://HONEYBEE.HELSINKI.FI/toothexp. Accessed October 2, 1999.

4 Tooth Enamel

LOCATION

Tooth enamel makes up the outside layer of the anatomic crown of a tooth. It covers and protects the dentin of the crown; follows the contours of the occlusal surface of a tooth; lines fissures, grooves, and pits; is firmly attached to the underlying dentin at the dentinoenamel junction; and meets the cementum at the cementoenamel junction (Fig. 4-1, see also Frontispiece).

Review the section on enamel formation in Chapter 3.

COMPOSITION

Enamel is composed of both inorganic (mineral) and organic substances. Mature human enamel is about 96% inorganic; the remaining 4% of its substance is an organic matrix (framework) and water. Enamel is the hardest tissue of the body; its mineral content far exceeds the mineral content of dentin (70%), cementum (50%), or bone (50%). Although considered a tissue of a tooth, enamel does not contain cells. Its formative cells (ameloblasts) do not become part of the enamel, and, in contrast to bone, enamel is devoid of blood vessels and nerves. Its structural unit is a rod composed of crystals. See Table 9-1 for a comparison of enamel to the other three mineralized tissues of the body.

MACROSCOPIC STRUCTURE OF ENAMEL

Examine the teeth of several persons who maintain reasonably good oral hygiene. The crown surfaces are composed of hard, shiny enamel. In young individuals who are free from dental caries, no other tooth tissues are exposed in the oral cavity. In older individuals, because of a normal aging process, the gingiva may have receded to such an extent that cementum is visible on some teeth. In persons of any age whose teeth have unrepaired caries lesions, dentin will be exposed in areas in which the disease has destroyed the enamel.

Numerous fine horizontal lines called perikymata[1] are usually seen on the enamel on the labial surfaces of the maxillary central incisors of a young person. In the cervical part of the crown, these lines are close together; incisally on the crown, they are farther apart (Fig. 4-2). Although perikymata are found on the enamel of

---

[1] Pronounced *pĕr ĭ kí mȧt ȧh.* peri (fr. Greek) = around; kymata (fr. Greek) = waves.

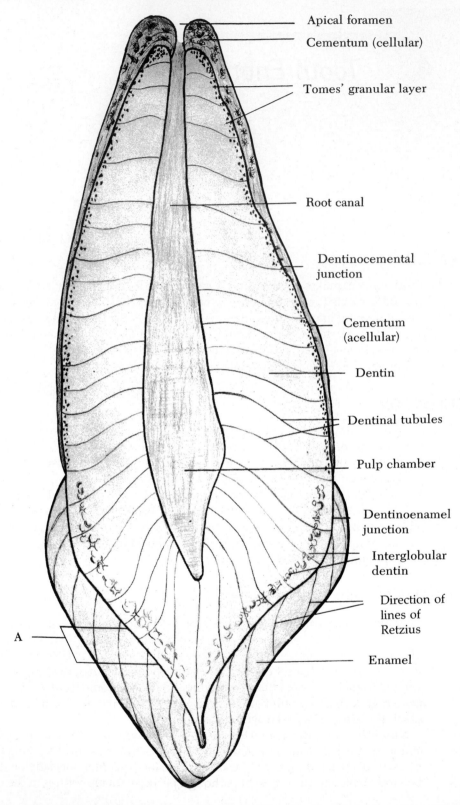

Apical foramen

Cementum (cellular)

Tomes' granular layer

Root canal

Dentinocemental junction

Cementum (acellular)

Dentin

Dentinal tubules

Pulp chamber

Dentinoenamel junction

Interglobular dentin

Direction of lines of Retzius

Enamel

A

Figure 4–1. Diagrammatic drawing of a longitudinal faciolingual section of a maxillary canine. The area marked A indicates a location in the enamel similar to that shown in Fig. 4-18.

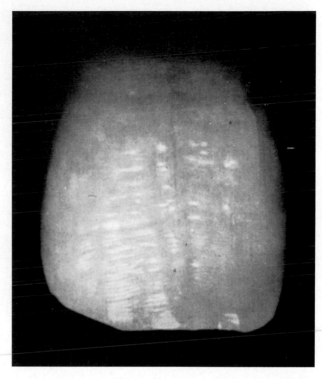

Figure 4–2. Labial surface of maxillary central incisor. The horizontal lines are perikymata.

all surfaces of all teeth, they are easier to see on more accessible surfaces. In older persons, perikymata usually are not visible and have been worn off of less protected surfaces.

As seen upon examination of their teeth, in older persons the enamel generally appears darker in color than in younger persons. Despite its hardness, tooth enamel is subject to *attrition*, that is, wearing off under the friction of use (see Fig. 1-13). Examine the teeth of several middle-aged persons. Usually the enamel of the molar cusps is worn so that the cusp tips are nearly flat. Sometimes the enamel is entirely worn off the cusp tips, and the exposed dentin is seen as dark spots (Fig. 4-3). In the anterior teeth, the incisal edges of the central and lateral incisors may be sufficiently worn to reveal dentin that is seen as a fine dark line extending mesiodistally on the incisal edge. These conditions of attrition in older individuals are not abnormal; they are merely a natural aging process. Accompanying changes in the dentin beneath the worn enamel protect the tooth pulp from damage (see Chapter 5).

Examine the newly emerged incisor teeth of a 6- or 7-year-old child. Three prominences, or scallops, are usually seen along the incisal edge. These prominences are developmental structures called mamelons[2] but are ordinarily of no clinical importance. Usually they are worn off early in the life of the tooth (Fig. 4-4).

Look carefully at the posterior teeth in an adult mouth and observe the *grooves* that mark the occlusal surface (Fig. 4-3). Grooves also are found on the buccal sur-

---

[2] Pronounced *măm ĕl ons*.

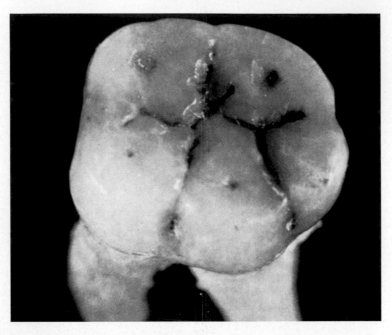

Figure 4–3. Attrition has almost exposed the dentin on the two buccal and two lingual cusps of this mandibular first molar. No apparent attrition is on the distal cusp. Notice the pits at the cervical ends of both the mesial and distal buccal grooves.

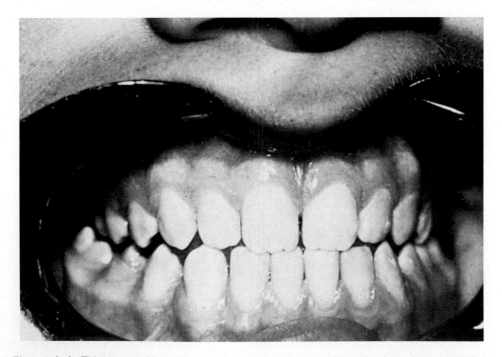

Figure 4–4. This young subject shows three incisal prominences (mamelons) on the two maxillary central incisors. Note that the mamelons of the left central are less pronounced, as wear has taken place.

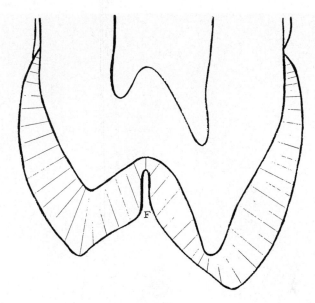

Figure 4–5. Diagrammatic drawing of a longitudinal faciolingual section of the crown of a maxillary first premolar tooth. The lines in the enamel illustrate the general direction of the enamel rods. Notice the narrowness of the fissure (F), the thinness of the enamel at the bottom of the fissure, and the radiating pattern of the enamel rods in the fissure.

faces of maxillary and mandibular molars (see Fig. 3-29), on the lingual surfaces of maxillary molars, on the lingual surfaces of the mandibular premolars, and sometimes on the lingual surfaces of maxillary and mandibular incisors. The depth of the grooves varies. In some teeth, they are shallow and smooth; in others, they are extended into deep *fissures* (Fig. 4-5, see also Frontispiece). On occlusal surfaces, the grooves and fissures may end in deep pits in the mesial and distal triangular fossae or in the central fossa. On the buccal and lingual surfaces, the grooves may have a deep pit at their cervical end. When examining the mouth, the depth of such fissures is impossible to determine, and usually the insertion of even the smallest dental instrument or toothbrush bristle into them is impossible (Figs. 4-5 and 4-6, see also Frontispiece). The pit and fissure do not extend into the dentin, but always end in the enamel. A small amount of enamel, however thin, always remains at the bottom of the pit or fissure and can be studied by examining ground sections of extracted teeth.

The enamel varies in thickness in different parts of the tooth crown. At its thickest parts, it may measure 2 or 2.5 mm, whereas at the cervical line, enamel may be only as thick as a knife-edge. Examine Figures 4-1 and 4-5 for an idea of the relative thickness of the enamel in different locations.

Enveloping the crown of the tooth and adhering firmly to its surface is the *enamel cuticle*, a covering that has been the subject of many studies since it was first described by Alexander Nasmyth in 1942. Although early histologists called this covering *Nasmyth's membrane*, it has been described in such diverse terms that it may seem as though not one, but several substances were being observed. For example, the enamel cuticle has been said to consist of cementum, denatured hemoglobin, and substances from saliva. However, because the nature of what

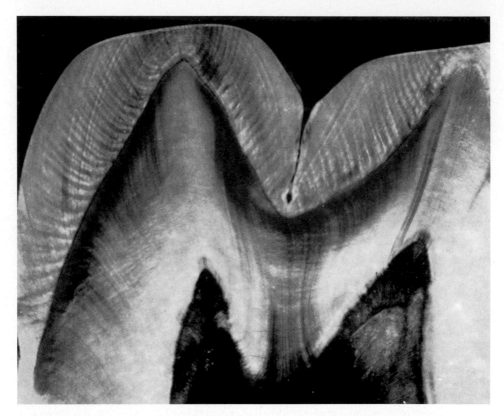

Figure 4–6. Ground section cut buccolingually through a mandibular molar. In the enamel, the dark and light bands of Hunter-Schreger extend from the dentinoenamel junction to the enamel surface nearly perpendicular to the dentinoenamel junction. The faintly visible lines of Retzius begin at the dentinoenamel junction and extend outward and occlusally, reaching the enamel surface, except near the cusp tip. In this tooth, some attrition is seen on the cusp tips. The magnification of this picture clearly shows that the fissure is too narrow to permit the insertion of any dental instrument. The enamel at the bottom of the fissure is thin and shows no sign of caries.

Nasmyth observed is unclear, the term enamel cuticle, rather than Nasmyth's membrane, is preferred.

Enamel cuticle is comprised of *primary enamel cuticle* and *secondary enamel cuticle*. Primary enamel cuticle is the last product of the enamel-forming ameloblasts (described in Chapter 3) and becomes mineralized. Secondary enamel cuticle is a product of the reduced enamel epithelium (also described in Chapter 3) and does not become mineralized. Secondary enamel cuticle (also called *dental cuticle*) is the outermost layer and most likely wears away after a period of tooth use. The dental cuticle is structurally described as a *basal lamina*, which is similar in appearance to the basal lamina of basement membranes found at the junction of epithelial and connective tissues (see Chapter 1).

MICROSCOPIC STRUCTURE OF ENAMEL

Enamel can be studied by various methods. An ordinary microscope allows for examination of thin ground sections of extracted teeth in their natural relationship with the organic and inorganic substances that constitute enamel. Or, the organic matrix, which is a delicate framework, can be examined separately using special careful techniques to dissolve away the mineral substances. Electron microscopy has enabled histologists to study enamel and other tissues at magnifications of the order of X5000 to X160,000.

Tooth enamel is made of minute rods or enamel prisms, each approximately 4 microns in diameter, that extend from the dentinoenamel junction toward the outer surface of the enamel. They are arranged roughly perpendicular to the dentinoenamel junction (Fig. 4-5) but are seldom perfectly straight and may contain multiple curvatures. A human maxillary central incisor contains approximately 8,586,000 enamel rods, and a maxillary first molar contains approximately 12,297,000 rods. Each enamel rod appears to be composed of a series of smaller units that resemble a string of beads (Figs. 4-7 and 4-8). This segmented construction is a result of the manner of formation of the rods.

Each enamel rod appears to be encased in a *rod sheath*, and the sheathed rods seem to be cemented together by an *inter-rod substance*. Of these structures, the rods are the most highly mineralized, followed by the cementing substance and rod sheaths. All three structures, however, are extremely hard. The organic substance that they contain has been shown by electron microscopy to exist as a fine fibrillar latticework of rods, rod sheaths, and inter-rod substance called the *organic matrix* of the enamel. In suitable preparations, this matrix may be examined with an ordinary microscope, but the fibrils of which it is composed are so minute that its fibrillar character can be seen only by the use of the electron microscope (Figs. 4-9, 4-10, 4-11, and 4-12).

The entire organic substance of enamel accounts for only 4% of its composition; the other 96% is mineral substance that exists as tightly packed *submicroscopic crys-*

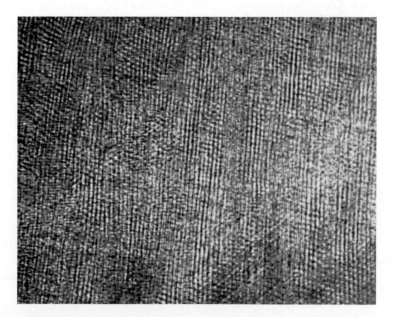

Figure 4–7. High-power photomicrograph of a ground section of human enamel. The rods extend from the dentinoenamel junction toward the tooth surface (from top to bottom of the picture) and in this area are nearly straight. The cross-striations in the rods are discernible.

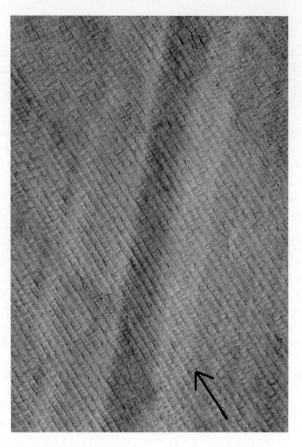

Figure 4–8. Higher magnification of enamel rods than those seen in Fig. 4-7. Inter-rod striations are clearly seen. The arrow indicates the direction of the rods.

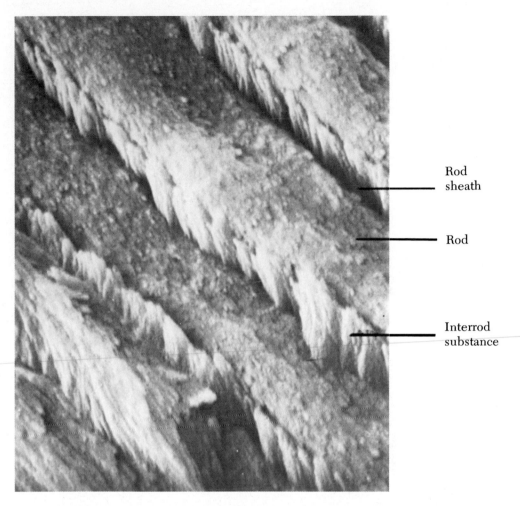

Rod
sheath

Rod

Interrod
substance

Figure 4–9. Scanning electron micrograph of freeze-fractured enamel of a deciduous central incisor (magnification X5250). Here, the arrangement and orientation of the apatite crystals can be seen. Note the tight packing of the rod crystals and their orientation along the long axis of the rods and, in the inter-rod areas, the slightly looser packing of the crystals and their almost perpendicular orientation to the rods. (Courtesy Dr. Ruth Paulson, College of Dentistry, Ohio State University.)

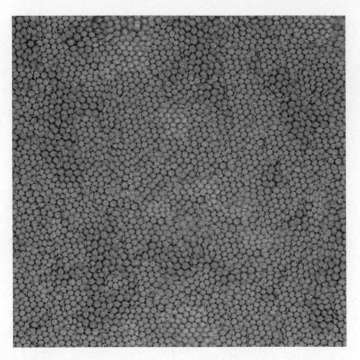

Figure 4–10. Cross section of enamel rods under light microscopy. Compare to Fig. 4-11, which is a view of enamel rods under electron microscopy.

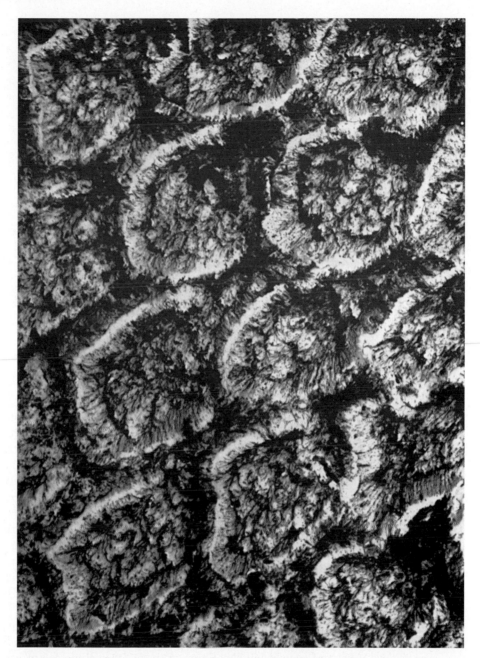

Figure 4–11. Electron micrograph of a shadowed replica of the end of enamel rods at the buccal surface of a mature human incisor. The clean enamel surface was first lightly acid-etched; then a softened nitrocellulose film was placed over the etched surface. When the dried film was removed, it carried the image of the etched surface. This film, called the replica, was shadowed at an angle of 40° with a palladium-and-gold alloy, which gave it contrast and a three-dimensional character by creating lights and shadows. The original magnification of the electron micrograph of the shadowed replica was X3,400.

This image is interpreted to be organic matrix of the enamel; most of the mineral substance was removed by the earlier acid-etching. The rods are seen in end-view, but there is no way of knowing how near to an exact cross section of the rods we are seeing. The broad white band around each rod conforms to the rod sheath, and the substance between the rods is interpreted as the inter-rod substance. (Courtesy Dr. Dennis Foreman, College of Dentistry, Ohio State University.)

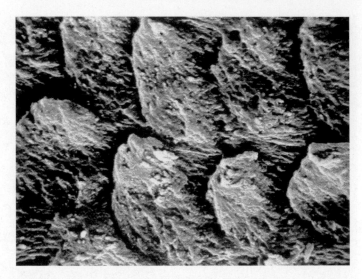

Figure 4–12. Scanning electron micrograph of enamel rods in cross section. Magnification is approximately X4,500. Note the fish-scale appearance of the rods. (Courtesy Dr. Ruth Paulson, College of Dentistry, Ohio State University.)

tals (Figs. 4-8, 4-11, and 4-12). These crystals fill the loose organic matrix and are so small that their size is measured in terms of millionths of a millimeter.

The chemical composition of the organic matrix of enamel has not been fully characterized, most likely because it is relatively unavailable for analysis and because of its close chemical bond to the inorganic material. Enamel contains two primary classes of protein, the *amelogenins* and the *enamelins*. Although their precise role in mineralization is unknown, they may regulate crystal formation by binding calcium or other components of hydroxyapatite.

The chemical nature of the inorganic part, which has been extensively studied, is generally agreed to be a crystalline calcium phosphate known as *hydroxyapatite*. In Figure 4-11, the electron micrograph of a replica of human enamel reveals rod outlines and the organic matrix of enamel. Most of the submicroscopic crystals have been dissolved by the acid-etching involved in specimen preparation. Figure 4-13 is a demineralized section of a developing tooth in which the enamel matrix was not fully mineralized. Consequently, the enamel was resistant to the action of the acid used during histologic preparation. It is referred to as acid-resistant enamel.

Examining a thin ground tooth section with an ordinary microscope reveals other formations in enamel: *bands of Hunter-Schreger*, *lines of Retzius*, *enamel lamellae*, *enamel tufts*, and *enamel spindles*. Some of these formations are of little known clinical importance, whereas others are of great importance.

When a longitudinal ground section of a tooth crown is examined under low-power light microscopy (Fig. 4-6), bands of Hunter-Schreger are seen as alternating broad light and dark bands. They extend perpendicularly from the dentino-enamel junction toward the tooth surface, and their manifestation results from the curvature of the enamel rods. In one band, the rods are oriented in longitudinal plane; in the adjacent band, as a result of rod curvatures, they are seen in transverse plane. This pattern can also be seen in a histologic section of a developing tooth that has been processed in such a way that the matrix of the forming enamel

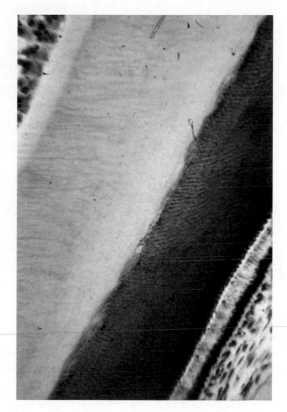

Figure 4–13. (See Color Plates) A demineralized section of an area of forming enamel and dentin. The dark-stained acid-resistant enamel lies adjacent to the lighter-stained dentin. Ameloblasts are seen along the enamel surface (lower right), and odontoblasts are along the pulpal surface of dentin (upper left).

has been retained. It also can be seen in specially prepared fully formed enamel examined under electron microscopy (Fig. 4-14). Admittedly, the pattern of curvature of a single rod is difficult to visualize.

The lines of Retzius are different kinds of bands in the enamel. In longitudinal ground sections of the tooth crown, they are seen under low-power light microscopy as narrow, brownish lines extending diagonally outward from the dentinoenamel junction toward the occlusal, or incisal, part of the crown (Figs. 4-1, 4-6, and 4-15). These lines are formed as a result of the layer-upon-layer pattern of enamel matrix formation and of the variations in structure and calcification along the lines corresponding to the formation pattern. On most of the crown, the lines of Retzius end on the crown surface, and their termination on the surface is marked by a series of shallow depressions. The ridges between the depressions are the perikymata. (This association between perikymata and the lines of Retzius is difficult to see in ground tooth sections.) Because the lines of Retzius do not reach the enamel surface near the incisal or occlusal part of the crown, there are no perikymata at the incisal edge or cusp tips. Perikymata often may be seen in clinical examination (Fig. 4-2).

Enamel lamellae (literally, *little layers*) are microscopic separations in the enamel that extend inward from the enamel surface for varying distances and are filled

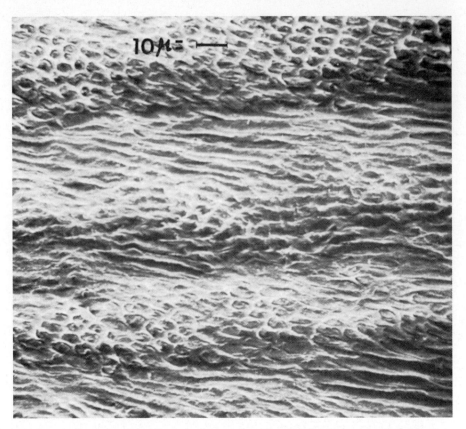

Figure 4–14. Bands of Hunter-Schreger in human enamel as seen with a scanning electron microscope. This freeze-fracture specimen from a premolar was taken from an area similar to the center of the crown on the left side of Fig. 4-10. Original magnification X450. (Courtesy Dr. Ruth Paulson, College of Dentistry, Ohio State University.)

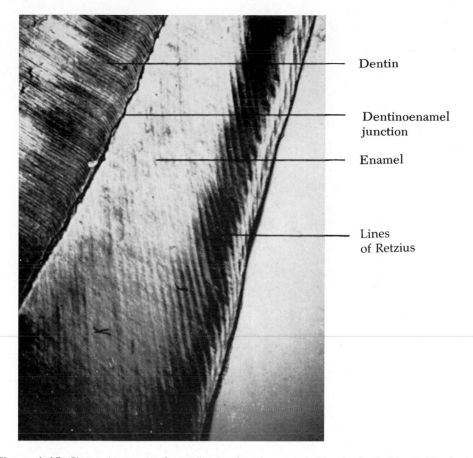

Dentin

Dentinoenamel
junction

Enamel

Lines
of Retzius

Figure 4–15. Photomicrograph of a small area of tooth crown, cut longitudinally. Lines of Retzius in the enamel are clearly visible. The direction of the dentinal tubules can also be seen. The occlusal surface is toward bottom of picture, the root toward the top.

with organic material (Figs. 4-16 and 4-17). They have been described by some histologists as faults in enamel matrix formation and by others as cracks in the enamel caused by injury.

Enamel tufts also are visible in ground tooth sections. Microscopically, they resemble small brushes that are attached to the dentinoenamel junction and extend outward in the enamel to as much as one fifth of the distance to the surface (Figs. 4-18 and 4-19). Histologically, they are the hypomineralized, or unmineralized, inner ends of some groups of enamel rods, rod sheaths, and surrounding inter-rod substance.

Enamel spindles are the peripheral ends of cytoplasmic processes of certain pulp cells (odontoblasts) that extend a short distance across the dentinoenamel junction into the enamel (Figs. 4-20 and 4-21). Their relationship with the dentin can be understood by studying the structure of dentin.

The dentinoenamel junction in many teeth is not a straight line, but a scalloped line in which small curved projections of enamel fit into small concavities of the dentin (Fig. 4-23).

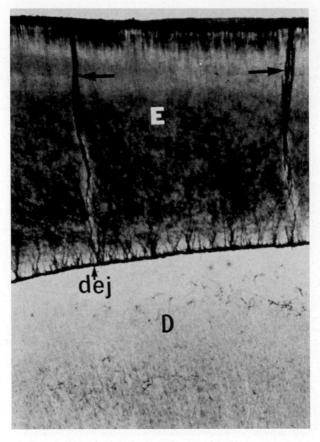

Figure 4–16. Photomicrograph of a ground section of a portion of a crown shows two enamel lamellae (arrows) extending from the surface into the enamel (E). DEJ, dentinoenamel junction; D, dentin.

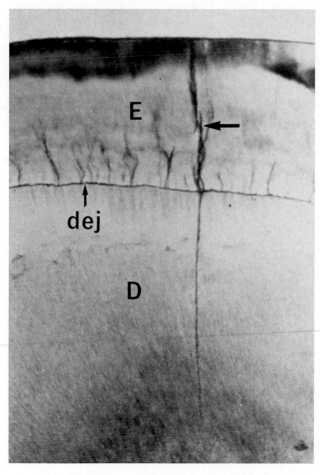

Figure 4–17. An enamel lamella (arrow) in this ground section extends from the enamel (E) surface, crosses the dentinoenamel junction (DEJ), and passes into the dentin (D).

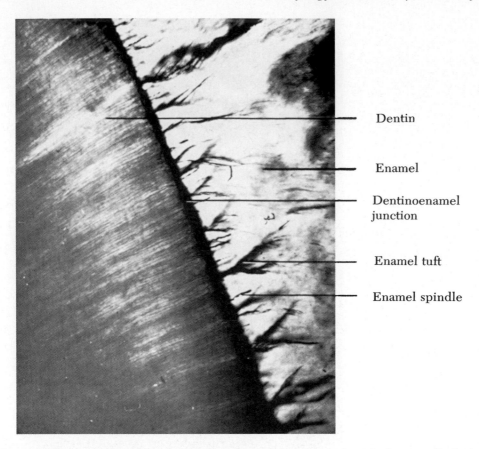

Dentin

Enamel

Dentinoenamel
junction

Enamel tuft

Enamel spindle

Figure 4–18. Photomicrograph of a small area of tooth crown, cut horizontally (low magnification). Among the clearly visible enamel tufts are the much smaller enamel spindles. See Fig. 4-18 for a higher magnification.

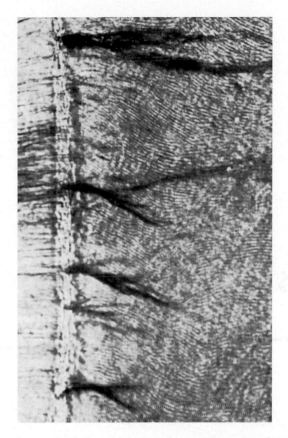

Figure 4–19. Photomicrograph of a ground section of enamel in an area of enamel tufts. This figure is a higher magnification of an area similar to that shown in Fig. 4-17.

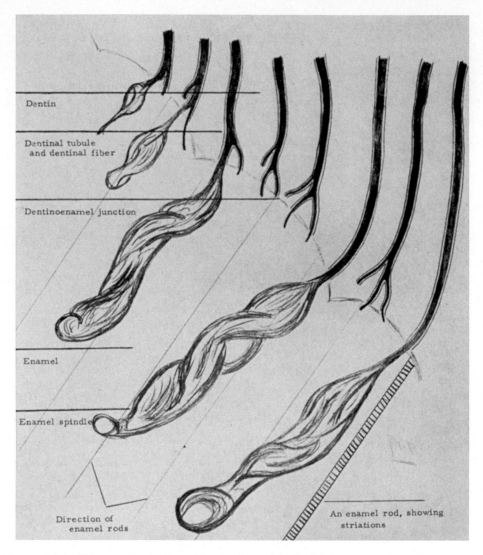

Figure 4–20. Diagrammatic drawing of details of area A in Fig. 4-1 shows enamel spindles.

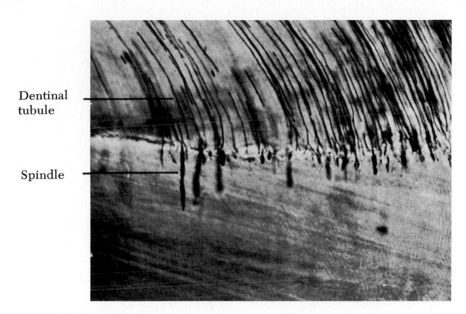

Figure 4–21. Photomicrograph of a ground section of a tooth crown near the cusp tip. Dentin is at the top of the picture; enamel is below. Many enamel spindles are seen in the enamel, and branching of the dentinal tubules is clear.

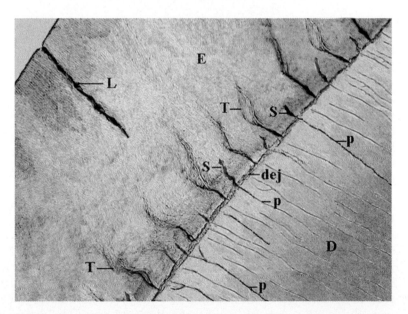

Figure 4–22. Composite view of enamel (E) structures. L, lamella originating at enamel surface; S, spindles arising from odontoblastic processes (P) of dentin (D), which cross the dentinoenamel junction (DEJ); T, tufts arising from the dentinoenamel junction.

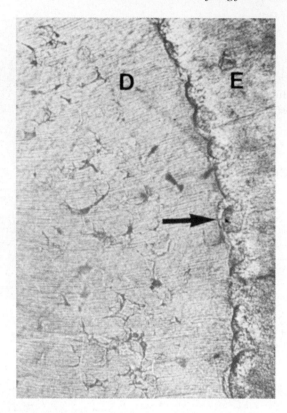

Figure 4–23. This ground section of an area of dentin (D) and enamel (E) is along the scalloped-appearing dentinoenamel junction (arrow).

Enamel contains no cells and is a product of specialized epithelial cells (ameloblasts). It has no circulation in the form of blood vessels or other structures, but its permeability to some substances has been demonstrated in studies using dyes and solutions of radioactive substances.

PERMANENCE OF ENAMEL

After tooth enamel is formed, the mineralization is never decreased by any cellular physiologic process within the tooth. Because the ameloblasts that form the enamel in the developing tooth are lost when the tooth emerges into the mouth, subsequent enamel formation is impossible. Therefore, enamel has only limited possibility of anatomic self-repair following damage by injury or by caries. There is, however, good evidence that the crystalline structure of surface enamel is in a state of dynamic flux with calcium and other minerals, such as fluoride, in the salivary fluids. This state of demineralization and remineralization is important in maintaining the integrity of the outer surfaces of enamel. The notion that pregnancy produces a physiologic withdrawal of calcium from the teeth of the mother is not supported by factual evidence.

CLINICAL IMPORTANCE OF THE STRUCTURE OF ENAMEL

Let us now consider how the character of tooth enamel may affect the clinical condition of the individual.

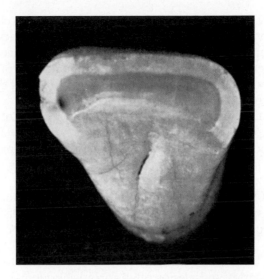

Figure 4–24. An extracted maxillary left central incisor photographed from the incisal aspect. The facial surface is toward the top. Attrition on the incisal edge has exposed the dentin. This edge was not ground off but is the result of wear from the friction of use. Notice the thickness of the enamel. The caries lesion visible in the dentin on the mesial (left) side began on the enamel surface around the mesial contact area. A diagonally-placed groove can be seen on the cingulum.

The high mineral content of enamel makes it a very hard substance that resists but is not immune to attrition during mastication (Figs. 4-3 and 4 6). On the incisal edges of anterior teeth and on the cusp tips of posterior teeth, where the teeth of opposing arches meet forcefully in occlusion, attrition may be sufficient to expose the underlying dentin (Figs. 4-24 and 4-25).

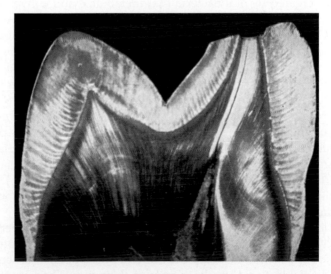

Figure 4–25. Ground section of a molar. The groove on the occlusal surface does not have a fissure at the bottom. No dental caries is present in the groove. Notice the direction of the dentinal tubules. The pulp horn extends far into the cusp (see Chapter 6).

The microscopic anatomy of enamel in many ways determines the strength and life of a tooth. Curvatures of the enamel rods increase its resistance to breakage, areas of low mineralization influence the pattern and speed of progress of caries, and the arrangement of the rods provides direction to the path of penetration of caries. Perikymata, which mark the enamel on all surfaces of the crown, are of no known clinical significance.

Bands of Hunter-Schreger, seen in ground sections of a tooth, are an optical phenomenon produced by curvatures in the enamel rods. These curvatures most likely reduce the chance of cleavage (splitting) of enamel along the rod length.

Enamel lamellae are believed by some investigators to be areas particularly susceptible to caries.

Lines of Retzius, areas of slightly less mineralization, to some degree facilitate the lateral spread of caries along each stripe. This spread, however, is considerably less pronounced than the lateral spread of caries that occurs at the dentinoenamel junction in areas of tufts and spindles.

Enamel tufts and spindles, which are hypomineralized areas, offer reduced resistance to caries, and a lesion often spreads horizontally in the enamel at the dentinoenamel junction. When the damaging agent enters the dentin, lateral spread of caries is still more extensive.

The arrangement of the enamel rods has an important influence on the pattern of penetration of caries in enamel, and the configuration of the dentinoenamel junction determines the pattern of arrangement of the rods.

DENTAL CARIES PROCESS

To understand the role of tooth structure in the occurrence and pattern of dental caries, one must understand the nature of this disease. Dental caries is a disease of the hard tissues of the teeth in which the mineral substance of the tooth is dissolved by acid, after which the organic substance is destroyed by proteolysis. The acid is created by oral bacteria that metabolize and convert carbohydrates, especially sugars, into acids. Caries-susceptible individuals have many of these acidogenic (acid-producing) bacteria in their saliva and dental plaques.

The bacteria that cause the damage are located in the *dental plaque*, a dense accumulation of microorganisms and salivary proteins that adhere firmly to the surface of a tooth. In mouths kept ordinarily clean, plaque is found chiefly in protected areas, around contact areas, and in pits and fissures (Fig. 4-26).

A known sequence of events follows the oral intake of sugar by a caries-susceptible person. Food taken into the mouth is retained in the area of the dental plaque covering the teeth. The acidogenic bacteria of the plaque then reduce the sugars to acids. Because the acids in the plaque are in contact with the tooth surface, the enamel beneath the plaque is slightly dissolved. This process is the beginning of a caries lesion. Repeated eating of sugar results in repeated periods of enamel dissolution.

The manner by which enamel is destroyed by acid is becoming better understood as studies with electron microscopy progress. The long, narrow submicroscopic crystals that make up the mineral phase of enamel seem to be most readily dissolved when acid attacks them from their ends. The crystals in the center of each rod are arranged with their long axes parallel to the long axis of the rod. Generally, the rods are arranged perpendicular to the dentinoenamel junction. The relation-

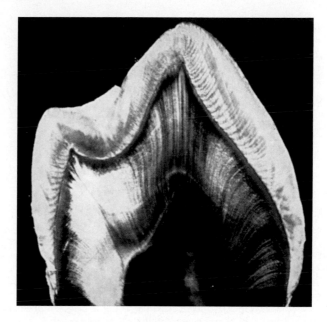

Figure 4–26. Ground section through a mandibular first premolar, cut buccolingually. The groove on the occlusal surface of the tooth is not deep, and no fissure is at the bottom. No caries is present in this groove, but a plaque is retained in the groove. Mineralized plaque is called calculus. Notice the direction of the dentinal tubules, which extend from the dentinoenamel junction to the pulp chamber (see Chapter 5).

ship of crystal orientation relative to the rod axes, the rod orientation relative to the dentinoenamel junction, and the configuration of the dentinoenamel junction determine the pattern of a caries lesion. The mechanism of dental caries continues to be under study, and answers presently accepted are subject to change as research progresses.

One recent change has been in the interpretation of white spot lesions. These areas of demineralization are localized in the enamel and thought to represent incipient carious lesions. Evidence indicates that these areas, when treated with fluoride and plaque control through good oral hygiene, can become remineralized such that the surface integrity of the enamel is restored.

SMOOTH SURFACE CARIES

Let us first consider a caries attack on the smooth facial, lingual, or proximal surface of a tooth. The dentinoenamel junction in these locations is straight or broadly convex; although the rods have curvatures, they extend toward the surface in a direction generally perpendicular to the dentinoenamel junction (see Fig. 4-1). Therefore, a lesion occurring around a contact area, for instance, penetrates more or less in a straight line toward the dentinoenamel junction.

PIT AND FISSURE CARIES

The grooves, fissures, and pits of the posterior teeth are particularly prone to caries. Although teeth without fissures and pits (Figs. 4-25 and 4-26) often, but not

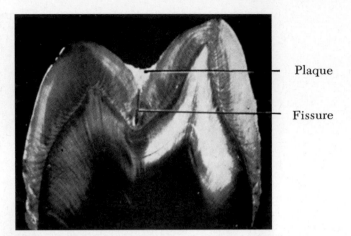

Figure 4–27. Ground section through a maxillary first premolar, cut buccolingually. The central groove has a deep fissure at its base. The thin enamel at the bottom of the fissure appears to be intact, but the appearance of the dentin immediately beneath it suggests that caries was present in the fissure at one side of the section seen here and that the lesion had spread near the dentinoenamel junction, thereby undermining the sound surface enamel. A dense plaque is present in the groove, but does not appear to be dense enough to be visible in the photomicrograph.

always, remain intact in their shallow grooves, teeth with fissures and pits provide an ideal environment for the growth of microorganisms. Although the fissure or pit may be so narrow and deep that even the smallest dental instrument cannot be inserted to the bottom (Figs. 4-6, 4-27, 4-28, and 4-29), it still permits the entrance of microorganisms and food into this sheltered, warm, moist, richly provided incubator, and a dental plaque can be expected to form here (Figs. 4-28 and 4-29). In a caries-susceptible person, when sugar is eaten and comes into contact with the plaque, acidogenic bacteria in the plaque create acid that damages the enamel walls of the pit or fissure, and caries result.

In occlusal fissures or pits, the form of a caries lesion is different from that of a smooth surface lesion. The enamel rods still lie nearly perpendicular to the dentinoenamel junction, but the sharp concavity of the junction in this location results in a radial pattern or fanning out of rods (Figs. 4-5 and 4-28). Microscopic examination of a tooth section rarely reveals a caries lesion at the bottom of a fissure that does not have an acute angle at the occlusal surface and a broad curved base at the dentinoenamel junction (Fig. 4-28). The result is a deceptive clinical picture. Clinical examination may reveal only a small carious area visible in a groove. However, at the dentinoenamel junction, invisible without radiographic images, the broadening of the lesion has left the surface enamel unsupported (Figs. 4-29 and 4-30).

Figure 4–29. Ground section of a molar. In this tooth, the caries began in the enamel at the bottom of the fissure and spread along the dentinoenamel junction. In this area, the lesion has visibly penetrated the dentin, and the effect of caries is seen in the dentin over a broad area of the dentinoenamel junction and pulpward. The dark region in the dentin beneath the fissure, broad near the dentinoenamel junction and more narrow nearer the pulp, is carious dentin (see Chapter 5). Caries spread downward, thereby destroying the unaffected dentin beneath and around it. Destruction of dentin leaves the superficial enamel unsupported.

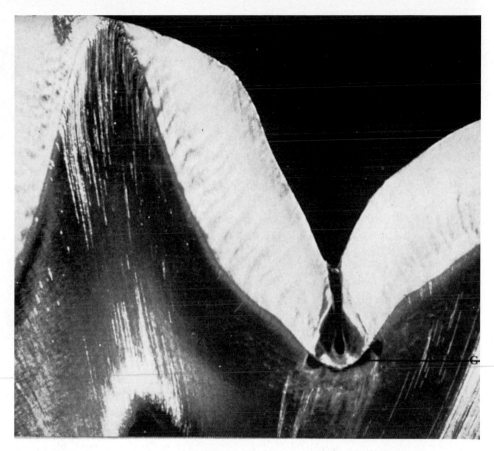

Figure 4–28. Ground section of a molar. The fissure in the occlusal groove clearly is affected by dental caries. Notice the radiating pattern of the lesion in the enamel near the bottom of the fissure. This pattern results from the fanning out of the enamel rods (see Fig. 4-5). The dentin beneath the bottom of the fissure is destroyed near the dentinoenamel junction (C), leaving the enamel unsupported. There is little evidence of sclerosis of the dentin beneath this lesion, and the bacteria here have probably penetrated well into the dentinal tubules (see Chapter 5). The plaque is indistinctly seen in this ground section. Often, plaques are destroyed in the process of grinding a specimen. Notice attrition on the cusp tip.

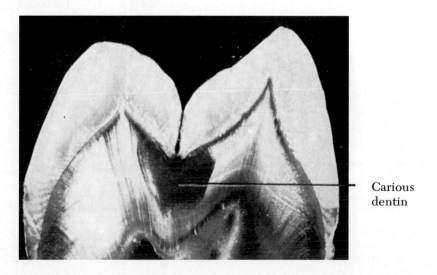

Carious dentin

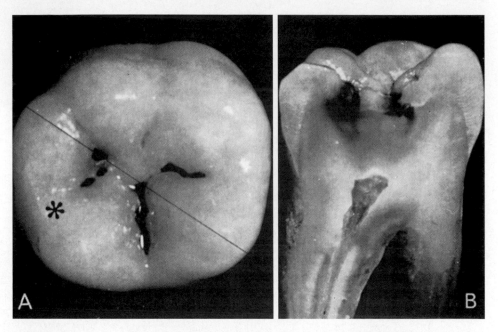

Figure 4–30. **A.** Even the casual observer can see that this mandibular first molar is carious in the occlusal fissures. The extent of the lesion is partly seen when the distolingual portion of the tooth (asterisk) is ground off. **B.** Caries had most likely penetrated to an area of the dentin beyond the cut surface seen here. Under the triangular ridge of the distal cusp, caries in the dentin has noticeably undermined the enamel.

Although fissures and pits are commonly thought of as occurring on occlusal surfaces of molar and premolar teeth, they are also found in other places. In some molar teeth, pits are found at the cervical end of buccal grooves (see Fig. 4-4). In Figure 4-31, the pit at the end of the buccal groove (Fig. 4-31A) has a caries lesion.

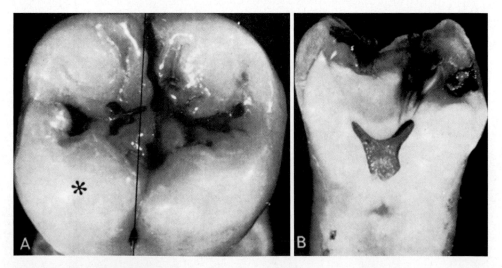

Figure 4–31. **A.** Caries is clearly seen in the occlusal grooves of this mandibular second molar. The buccal pit at the end of the buccal groove (bottom of picture) appears to be deep but undamaged. **B.** Removal of the mesial side of the tooth (asterisk in A) reveals considerable caries damage in the buccal pit and a deep penetration into the occlusal dentin beneath the bucco-occlusal groove.

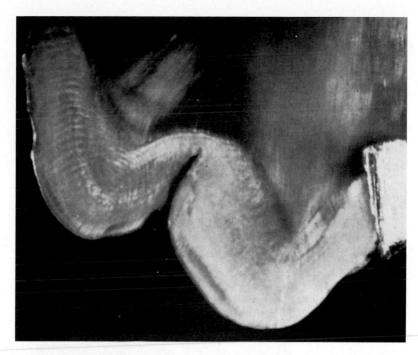

Figure 4–32. A maxillary first molar with a prominent cusp of Carabelli was ground to reveal the deep fissure at the line of attachment of this fifth cusp of the mesiolingual cusp. In this tooth, the enamel of the fissure appears to be intact. In some similar fissures, caries is present. The cusp of Carabelli is at the left of the picture. The oblong object at the right is part of an amalgam filling in the occlusal surface.

Although the lesion is not apparent from the outside, it penetrates some distance into the dentin (Fig. 4-31B).

At the junction of the cusp of Carabelli and at the mesiolingual cusp of a maxillary molar to which it is attached, there is a groove, often deep enough to be called a fissure, that is susceptible to caries (Fig. 4-32).

Unexpectedly, a pit may be present at the incisal border of the cingulum of a maxillary incisor that has a deep lingual fossa and heavy marginal ridges (Fig. 4-33). A ground section of this tooth reveals a deep developmental depression. When such an invagination is so deep that it protrudes into the pulp cavity, it is called a *dens in dente* (a tooth in a tooth). Notice that enamel lines the surface of this invagination.

In some mongoloid peoples, deep, apicoincisally oriented grooves occur characteristically on the cingulum of mandibular incisors. In such places, caries often develops.

Surprisingly, pits often are on the incisal edges of mandibular incisor teeth when prominent mamelons are present. The pits seen in Figure 4-34 are not carious, but sometimes in such pits early caries can be detected in the study of a ground section.

These structural characteristics of enamel that tend to facilitate the spread of caries beneath the enamel surface can explain how biting on something firm can cause part of the surface of what appears to be a good tooth to cave in. An understanding of the subsurface spread of dental caries motivates the dentist and the dental hygienist to instruct patients on the importance of regular dental examinations and the necessity for prompt attention to even seemingly small cavities.

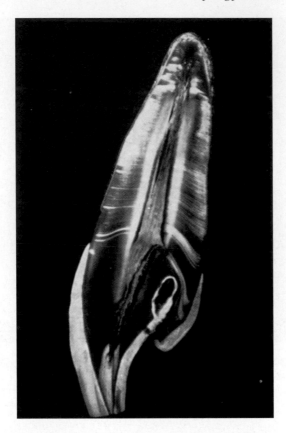

Figure 4–33. This maxillary central incisor had a deep lingual fossa, pronounced marginal ridges, and what appeared to be a pit at the incisal border of the cingulum. It was ground to a thin center section. In this photomicrograph, what appeared to be a small lingual pit is seen to extend into the tooth and to be lined with a thin layer of enamel. No caries was evident in this tooth, even when the section was examined under high magnification. However, caries frequently is found in such invaginations, and in some teeth this kind of developmental invagination is much deeper and is called dens in dente (tooth within a tooth).

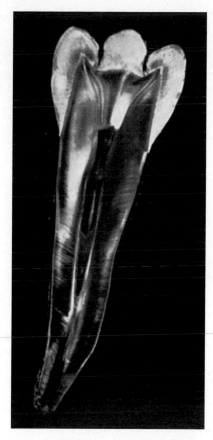

Figure 4–34. Ground section of mandibular incisor, cut mesiodistally. The intact tooth had mamelons that appeared unusually pronounced. The ground section shows deep pits in the depressions between the mamelons, with a thin layer of enamel at the bottom of the pits. In ground sections of several teeth that had unusually pronounced mamelons, such pits were generally present. Notice the curvature of the dentinal tubules in the tooth crown. In the root, the tubules are nearly straight and are directed slightly apically from the cementodentinal junction.

AGE-RELATED CHANGES

Enamel undergoes changes with age. Some of the changes are clinical observations; others are supported by scientific data.

The most common age-related change of enamel is attrition—the wearing away of tooth substances as a result of mastication. Cusp tips and incisal edges may wear away completely, thereby exposing the dentin. Excessive wear may also lead to the elimination of pits and fissures.

Other age-related changes of enamel are decreased permeability, darker color, reduction of caries, and increase of fluoride content at the surface. Many of these changes are associated with the eating habits and environment of the individual.

SUGGESTED READINGS

Carranza FA Jr. Glickman's clinical periodontology. 7th Ed. Philadelphia: W.B. Saunders; 1990.
Fejerskov O, Ekstrand J, Burt BA. Fluoride in Dentistry. Copenhagen: Munksgaard, 1996

Newbrun E, ed. Fluorides and Dental Caries: Contemporary concepts for practitioners and students. 3rd Ed. Springfield (IL): Thomas, 1986.

Newbrun E. Cariology. 3rd Ed. Chicago: Quintessence Publishing Co., 1989.

Smith CE. Cellular and chemical events during enamel maturation. Crit Rev Oral Biol Med 1998;9:128–161.

Zhou R, Zaki AE, Eisenmann DR. Morphometry and autoradiography of altered rat enamel protein processing due to chronic exposure to fluoride. Arch Oral Biol 1996;41:739–747.

5   Dentin

LOCATION

Dentin is located in both the crown and roots of a tooth, making up the bulk of the tooth. It encloses and is intimately associated with the tooth pulp. Tooth pulp is a soft connective tissue that forms an interdependent complex with the hard dentin. In an intact tooth the dentin is not visible because in the crown it is covered by enamel and in the root by cementum (Figs. 5-1 and 5-2).

Review the section on dentin formation in Chapter 3.

COMPOSITION

Like all mineralized tissues of the body, dentin is composed of both *organic* (protein) and *inorganic* (mineral) substances. Although not nearly as hard as tooth enamel, dentin is harder than cementum and bone. Mature dentin is about 70% inorganic substance and about 30% organic material and water. (Compare these figures to those given for enamel in Chapter 4.)

STRUCTURE OF DENTIN

The organic part of dentin, known as the organic matrix, is composed of small fibrils and a surrounding, structureless *ground substance*. During dentin development, the organic matrix is formed first; then minerals in solution, similar to the minerals of enamel, cementum, and bone, are deposited in the cementing substance (see Table 9-1). Dentin becomes a hard tissue when the minerals crystallize out of solution and form on and around the fibrils.

The organic matrix of dentin consists of *collagen* fibrils and a ground substance of glycosaminoglycans. The inorganic material consists of hydroxyapatite crystals, as in enamel, cementum, and bone.

Dentin is perforated by innumerable channels, called *dentinal tubules*, each of which contains a cell process. The tubules lie close together and extend from the tooth pulp to the dentinoenamel junction in the crown of the tooth and to the dentinocemental junction in the root (Figs. 5-2 and 5-3). At their outer ends, the dentinal tubules are divided into numerous branches (Fig. 5-4). Much smaller branches connecting adjacent dentinal tubules are often found along the length of the tubules. The dentinal tubules measure approximately 3 microns in diameter at

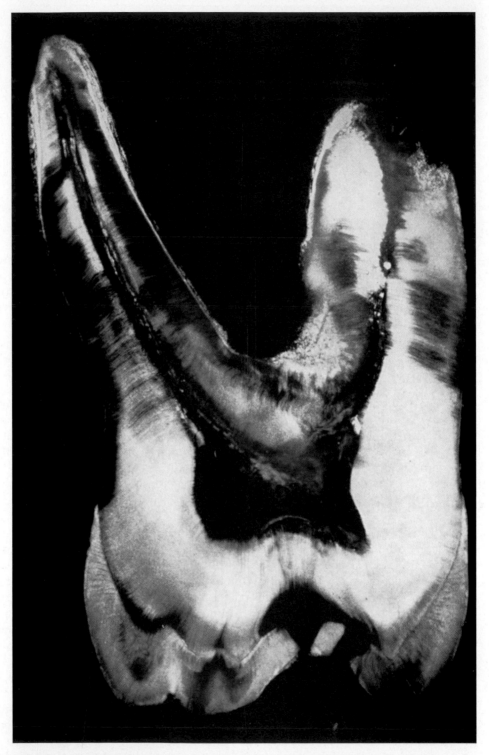

Figure 5–1. Photomicrograph of a ground section through a maxillary first molar, cut buccolingually. This tooth is shown diagrammatically in Fig. 5-2.

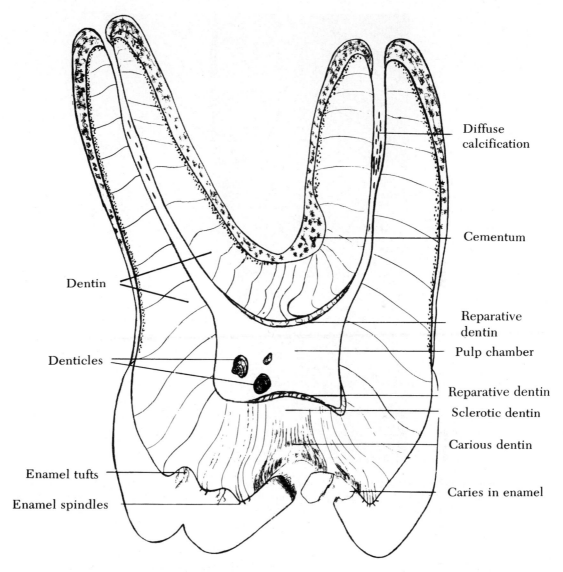

Labels on figure: Diffuse calcification, Cementum, Reparative dentin, Pulp chamber, Reparative dentin, Sclerotic dentin, Carious dentin, Caries in enamel, Dentin, Denticles, Enamel tufts, Enamel spindles

Figure 5–2. Diagrammatic drawing of a longitudinal buccolingual section of a maxillary first molar. Dental caries has destroyed the enamel in the area around a groove on the occlusal surface. The caries has spread horizontally at the dentinoenamel junction and undermined the enamel. Caries has spread pulpward in the dentinal tubules to about two thirds the thickness of dentin. The dentin close to the pulp is sclerotic dentin; the tubules are filled with mineral salts. On the pulpal wall beneath the caries lesion, a small amount of reparative dentin has formed. The reparative dentin on the floor of the pulp chamber (next to the root) was not caused by caries; reparative dentin in this location is not unusual. (See Fig. 5-1.)

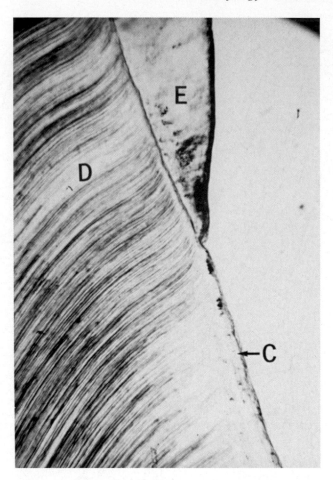

Figure 5–3. Ground section of the cervical part of a tooth shows relation of the dentinal tubules (D) to the enamel (E) and cementum (C). The tubules appear dark here. Because of processing, the tubules are filled with air.

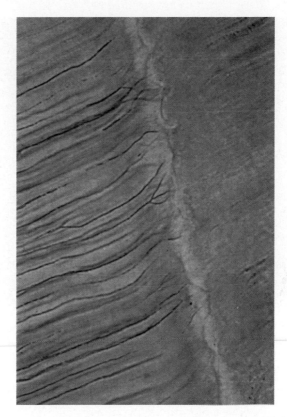

Figure 5–4. Microscopic section cut along the dentinoenamel junction (lighter diagonal layer); enamel is on the left, dentin on the right. The dentinal tubules, with their contained cell processes, branch at their outer ends along the dentinoenamel junction. The odontoblastic cell processes within the tubules appear to be fibrils because of the shrinkage of the processes during histologic preparation.

the pulpal ends and somewhat less at the other ends (Figs. 5-5, 5-6, 5-7, and 5-8). In the cusp area in the tooth crown and in the apical half of the root, the dentinal tubules are nearly straight and are arranged nearly perpendicular to the dentinoenamel or dentinocemental junctions. In the facial, lingual, mesial, and distal areas of the crown and in the cervical portion of the roots, the dentinal tubules are S-shaped. The outer ends of the S-shaped tubules are always occlusal to the pulpal ends of the tubules (Figs. 5-2 and 5-3). The thin sheath of *peritubular dentin* that surrounds each dentinal tubule has a higher mineral content and lesser organic content than the remaining intertubular dentin.

A cell process—the cytoplasm extension of a pulp cell—occupies each dentinal tubule (see Figs. 4-21, 5-8, 5-9, and 5-10). The cells of the pulp that lie next to the dentin have the somewhat surprising distinction of also being dentin cells. They are named *odontoblasts* and form the *organic matrix* of dentin. They also serve to provide nutrition to dentin and possibly play a role in the pain sensation of a tooth. The nucleus of the odontoblast cell remains in the pulp, surrounded by part of the cytoplasm of the cell body. The remainder of the cytoplasm of the odontoblast cell is stretched out like a long, thin tail and extends into a dentinal tubule (see Figs. 3-21 and 5-10). This cytoplasmic extension of the odontoblast is the *odontoblastic pro-*

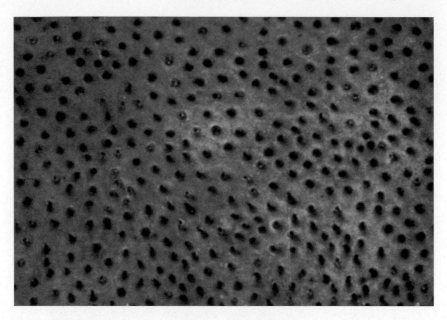

Figure 5–5. Photomicrograph of a ground section of dentin cut to reveal the dentinal tubules in cross section. The specimen was dipped in a histologic stain that remained in the tubules, making them appear dark in the picture. The tubules in this section, taken from near the tooth pulp rather than close to the enamel, are approximately 3 mm in diameter.

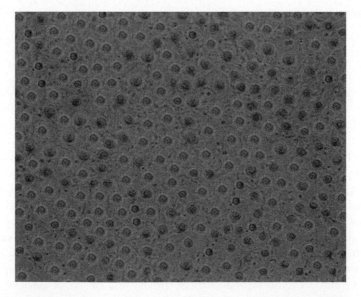

Figure 5–6. Cross section of the dentinal tubules with enclosed odontoblastic processes. Sites of *peritubular* dentin (walls of the tubules), the hardest and most mineralized part of the dentin, are the distinct clear-stained areas around the odontoblastic processes.

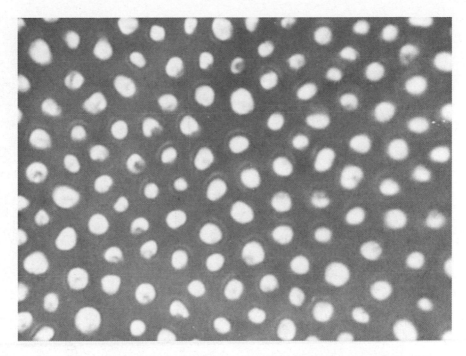

Figure 5–7. Cross section of the dentinal tubules. This demineralized specimen is at a higher magnification than that seen in Fig. 5-5. Most of the tubules are empty; some contain shrunken odontoblastic processes.

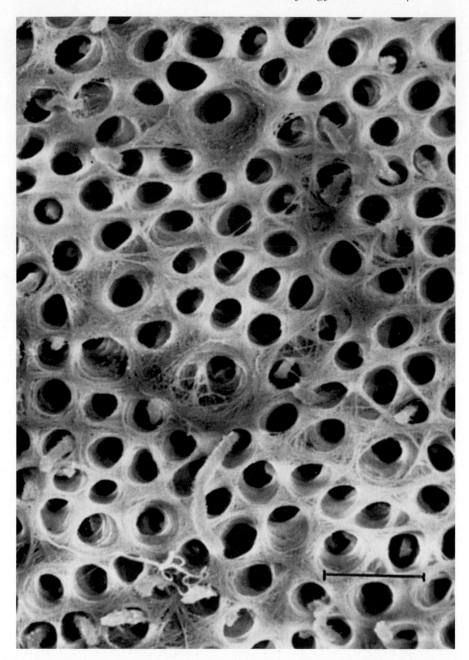

Figure 5–8. Scanning electron micrograph of the cross section of dentinal tubules adjacent to the pulp chamber of a human tooth. Odontoblastic processes can be seen in some of the orifices. The black line engraved in the lower right measures 10 μm. (Courtesy Dr. Dennis Foreman, College of Dentistry, Ohio State University.)

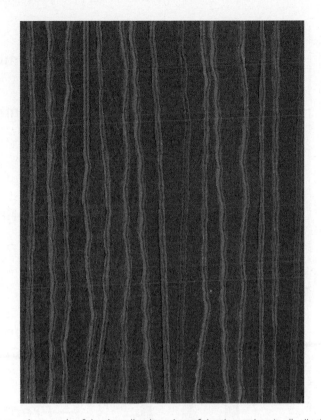

Figure 5–9. Photomicrograph of demineralized section of dentin, cut longitudinally through the dentinal tubules. Odontoblastic processes can be identified within the tubules.

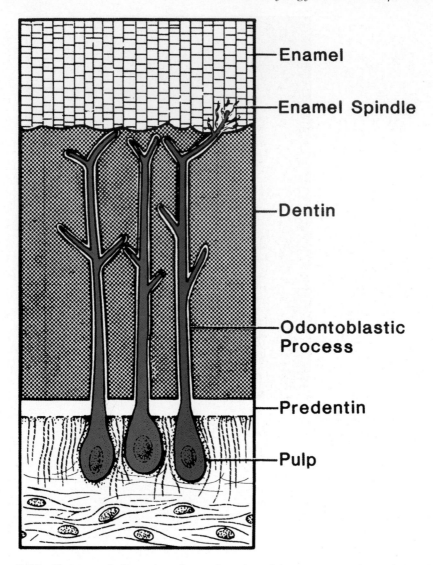

Figure 5–10. Diagrammatic illustration of a small portion of the crown area shows three odontoblasts. The cell body (nuclear part) of the odontoblast lies in the pulp, and its process extends into the dentinal tubule. Notice the branching of the processes and the entrapped end of a process (an enamel spindle) within the enamel.

cess. In young teeth, each process extends through the tubule to the dentinoenamel or dentinocemental junction. At their peripheral ends, the processes are branched just as the tubules are branched (see Figs. 4-21, 5-4, and 5-10). In older teeth, the processes apparently are withdrawn and are found only in the pulpal ends of the tubules.

In some places in the crown of a tooth, the peripheral ends of some odontoblastic processes cross the dentinoenamel junction and protrude into the enamel. Here, they appear as short, slightly thickened objects. These ends of processes in the enamel, or the empty spaces once occupied by ends of the processes, are enamel spindles (see Figs. 4-20, 4-21, and 5-10).

Adjacent to the pulp, young teeth always have a layer of dentin that is less mineralized than the rest of the dentin. This layer is called *predentin* or *dentoid* and is actually the organic matrix of dentin that has not yet mineralized. Figure 5-11 is a photomicrograph of a section cut through the root of a young tooth that was demineralized and prepared for histologic viewing. Predentin is clearly visible in this section. Because it is less mineralized, predentin stains lighter than mineralized dentin. Predentin also indicates the incremental (layer upon layer) or appositional pattern by which dentin is formed; as a result, growth lines, called *von Ebner* lines, are seen in the mineralized dentin (Fig. 5-12).

In the crowns of some teeth, the dentin contains spots that are unmineralized or are hypomineralized (hypo = under, less than ordinary). These unmineralized spots are irregular in shape and usually occur in a layer a short distance inside the

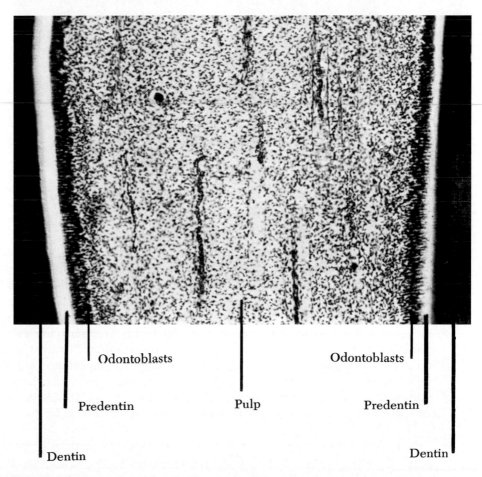

Odontoblasts   Odontoblasts

Predentin   Pulp   Predentin

Dentin   Dentin

Figure 5–11. Microscopic view of a young tooth section (cut through the root) shows the odontoblast cell layer, the predentin layer, and the dentin on each side of the pulp tissue. Notice the striking contrast between the unmineralized predentin and the mineralized dentin. Because predentin and dentin differ chemically, they stain differently when processed for histologic viewing. The densely packed dots scattered throughout the pulp are nuclei of cells, most of which are fibroblasts. The dark fibrillar structures among the cells are blood vessels and nerves.

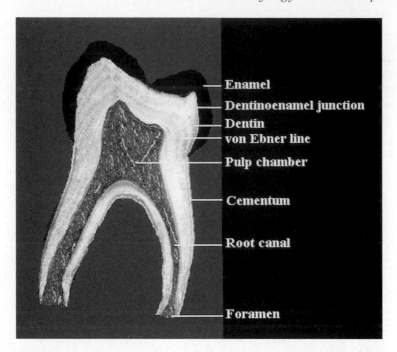

Figure 5–12. Histologic section of a primary molar showing von Ebner lines (incremental or appositional growth lines in dentin).

dentinoenamel junction (see Figs. 4-1, 5-13, and 5-14). In this location, such an area of unmineralized dentin—called *interglobular dentin*—surrounds areas of *globular dentin* that have a normal mineral content (Figs. 5-14 and 5-15). Failure of proper mineralization in this location is believed to be a result of a metabolic disturbance that occurred during formation of this part of the tooth.

Root dentin invariably contains a band of minute unmineralized spots almost immediately beneath the cementum. This band, called *Tomes' granular layer* (see Figs. 4-1, 5-16, and 5-17), was first described by the dental histologist Sir John Tomes (1815–1895), who thought that this region of the dentin had a granular appearance. Subsequent investigation revealed that this area is not really granular, but is made of small unmineralized spots in the dentin. There is evidence that these granular spots are produced by looping of the terminal portions of dentinal tubules. Tomes' granular layer has considerable clinical importance, which will be reviewed later. In the root dentin of some teeth, a short distance beneath Tomes' granular layer, a layer of interglobular dentin may exist which is similar in size and configuration to the interglobular dentin found in the crown of the tooth (Fig. 5-16).

A modified type of dentin known as *reparative dentin* is usually found along the pulpal wall of older teeth. Although its dentinal tubules are fewer and less regular than those of the first dentin produced, reparative dentin is similar to the earlier dentin. Reparative dentin may be formed throughout the life of the tooth as long as the pulp is healthy and is sometimes referred to as *secondary dentin* by dental clinicians. Reparative dentin produced in response to attrition, caries, operative procedures, or other damaging stimuli usually has fewer and more irreg-

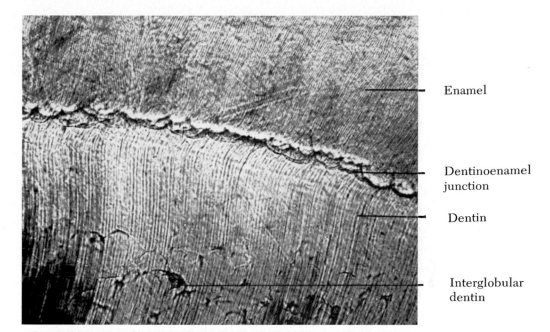

Figure 5–13. Photomicrograph of part of a ground section of a tooth crown. The enamel is attached to the dentin at the scalloped dentinoenamel junction. Curvatures in the enamel rods are evident, and in some areas cross-striations of the rods can be seen. In the dentin at the bottom of the picture are irregular (dark) areas of interglobular dentin.

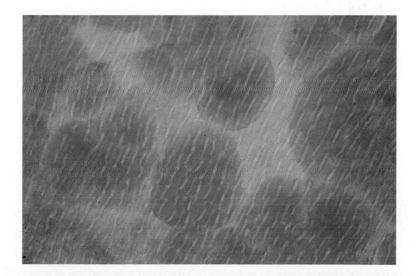

Figure 5–14. (See Color Plates) Microscopic view of a demineralized section of crown dentin, cut through areas of interglobular dentin. The dark-stained globular areas are mineralized; the lighter-stained irregularly shaped areas of interglobular dentin are unmineralized. Note that parts of dentinal tubules are found throughout globular and interglobular areas. Compare to the ground section in Fig. 5-13.

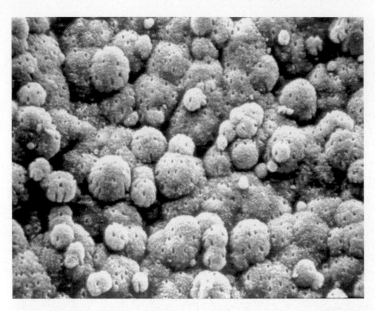

Figure 5–15. This scanning micrograph clearly shows the globular formation pattern of dentin. Interglobular dentin occurs between the globules (clear areas in Fig. 5-14). The small pores are dentinal tubules. (Courtesy of Dr. Ruth Paulson, College of Dentistry, Ohio State University.)

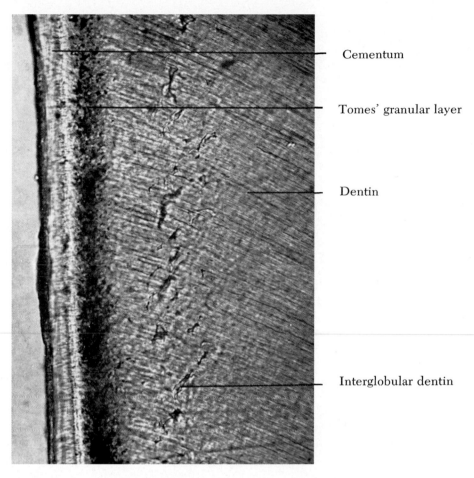

Cementum

Tomes' granular layer

Dentin

Interglobular dentin

Figure 5–16. Photomicrograph of part of a ground section of tooth root, high power magnification. The cementum is the relatively narrow light band (left); the dentin is the wide area (right). In the dentin and close to the cementum is the band of closely packed areas of uncalcified dentin called Tomes' granular layer. Deeper in the dentin are larger, irregular areas of interglobular dentin (dark areas). Notice that the dentinal tubules are straight and at right angles to the cementodentinal junction. The small lines perpendicular to the cementum surface are spaces once occupied by Sharpey's fibers (see Chapter 7). Was the crown of this tooth located beyond the top or beyond the bottom of this picture?

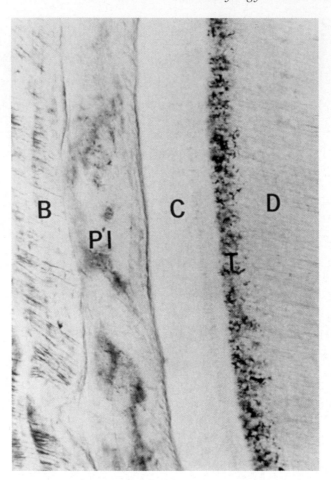

Figure 5–17. Microscopic view of a ground section of a portion of a tooth root and its surrounding tissues. The less mineralized and granular-appearing Tomes' granular layer (T) is clearly seen within the outer surface of the root dentin (D), next to the conspicuous acellular cementum (C). The periodontal ligament (PL) is well delineated between the cementum and bone (B) of the tooth socket. Because this example is a ground section, cellular detail of the bone and periodontal ligament is lacking.

ular dentinal tubules than dentin produced merely as a result of aging. Dental clinicians sometimes use the term secondary dentin when referring to reparative dentin.

Figure 5-18 is a histologic section of dentin taken from a tooth that functioned in the oral cavity for several years after an operative procedure had been performed to place a filling. The section extends from the cut surface to the pulp. Beneath the surface is a dead tract where the dentinal tubules are void of cell processes and are darkened because of the air in the empty tubules. On the pulp side of the dead tract is an area of reparative dentin that protrudes into the pulp and is strikingly different from the rest of the dentin. It has fewer dentinal tubules and has a glassy appearance that results from its higher content of mineral salts.

In certain areas on the pulpal wall, reparative dentin is formed in larger amounts. In posterior teeth, it is formed in larger amounts on the floor of the pulp chamber and in the pulp horn, which extends toward the cusp tips (Figs. 5-2, 5-18,

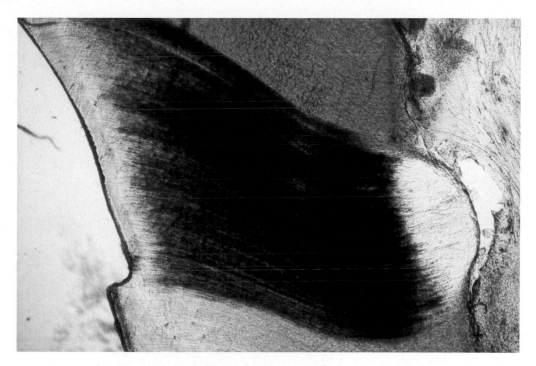

Figure 5–18. (See Color Plates) Microscopic view of an area of dentin beneath a surface (left) that was cut to receive a filling. Clearly visible is a dead tract, where the dentinal tubules are void of cell processes and are darkened because of the presence of air. Pulpal to the dead tract is a clear area of reparative dentin protruding into the pulp cavity on the right.

5-19, and 5-20). In anterior teeth, reparative dentin forms in larger amounts beneath the incisal edge when there has been considerable attrition (see Figs. 4-1, 5-19, and 5-21), or it may occur in larger amounts on the pulpal wall where dental caries has penetrated to the dentinoenamel junction (Figs. 5-1, 5-2, and 5-22). Its greater formation in these areas is often a result of the reaction of tooth pulp to the irritation of attrition or caries.

Sclerotic dentin is a modified dentin frequently found in old teeth and less frequently in young teeth. Dentin is sclerotic when the odontoblastic processes have withdrawn and the dentinal tubules have become filled with calcium salts. When peritubular dentin continues to form, the diameter of the dentinal tubule progressively decreases, and the resistance across the dentin increases. Therefore, it is more difficult for toxic substances and bacteria to move from the oral cavity to the dental pulp.

In the mandibular incisor tooth shown in Figure 5-21, the odontoblastic processes have degenerated beneath the worn incisal edge, but the dentinal tubules have not become filled with calcium salts. Such an area has been referred to as a *dead tract*. The pulp beneath the dead tract in this tooth is protected by the presence of reparative dentin. At the cervix on the facial side of this tooth, a change in the dentin has occurred beneath the cervical abrasion. The white area, indicated by the pointer, is probably a dead tract. Outside the dead tract, nearer the surface of the

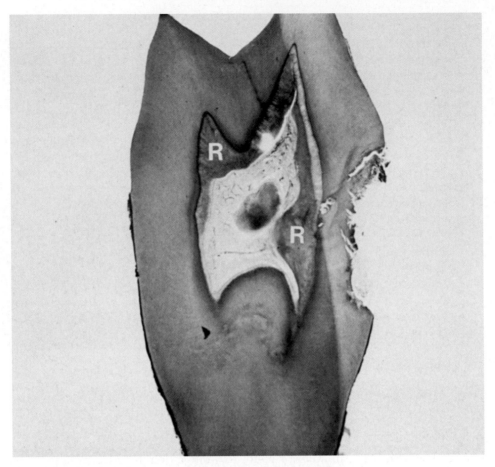

Figure 5–19. Microscopic view of a demineralized tooth shows reparative dentin (R) in the horns of the pulp chamber and under the caries (right). The structure surrounded by pulp tissue is a pulp stone. The root canal is not seen because the tooth was sectioned at an angle and the enamel was lost during histologic processing.

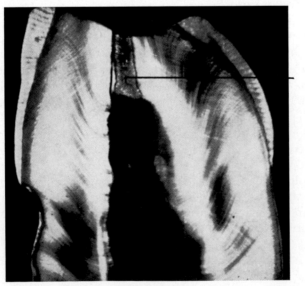

Reparative dentin

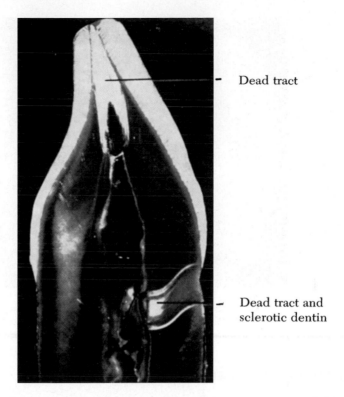

Dead tract

Dead tract and sclerotic dentin

Figure 5–21. Photomicrograph of a ground section of a mandibular incisor, cut faciolingually. Beneath the worn incisal edge is a dead tract in the dentin. Deposition of reparative dentin beneath the dead tract has protected the pulp from damage. On the facial side of the tooth in the cervical area is abrasion. The cementum is gone, and some of the dentin has been worn away. Beneath this abraded surface is an alteration in the dentin. Near the pulp is an area of dead tract, which appears white. Superficial (nearer the surface) to this tract, the dentin appears sclerotic. On the pulp wall in this region, reparative dentin has been produced and protrudes into the pulp cavity inside the dead tract. Notice the curvature of the dentinal tubules in the cervical area.

tooth, the dentin appears to be sclerotic, and the tubules are filled, or are becoming filled, with calcium salts.

Sclerotic dentin is often found beneath worn enamel, such as occurs in the incisal area of anterior teeth, and beneath slowly progressing dental caries where reparative dentin is being produced on the pulpal wall (Figs. 5-2 and 5-21). Sclerotic dentin is also found beneath Tomes' granular layer in the cervical area of older teeth where the cervical cementum has become exposed to the oral cavity as a result of gingival recession (see Chapter 11).

Figure 5–20. Photomicrograph of a ground section of a canine tooth, cut faciolingually. Extensive attrition has resulted in the loss of the enamel and part of the dentin of the cusp. The formation of reparative dentin in the incisal part of the pulp cavity has protected the pulp from exposure.

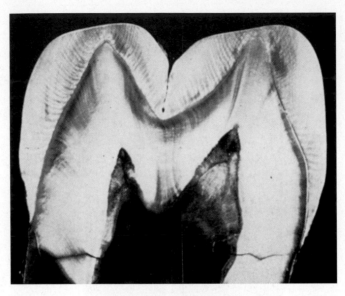

Figure 5–22. Photomicrograph of a ground section of a mandibular molar. A large amount of reparative dentin has formed in the pulp horns of both the buccal and lingual cusps. Notice the attrition of the enamel on the cusp tips.

CLINICAL IMPORTANCE OF DENTINAL STRUCTURE

The structure of dentin influences both the pattern of a carious lesion and the speed with which dental caries destroys a tooth. Structure also accounts for the sensitivity frequently experienced by patients during the performance of an oral prophylaxis or the eating of hot or cold foods.

In the preceding chapter, dental caries was explained as a disease of the hard tissues of the tooth. Acidogenic bacteria convert sugars into acids that dissolve the minerals of the hard tooth tissues, and proteolytic (proteo = protein; lytic = destroying) bacteria destroy the organic component of the hard tooth tissue in the same area.

When the caries process penetrates the enamel as far as the dentinoenamel junction, the caries-producing bacteria also reach this depth and come in contact with the peripheral ends of the dentinal tubules. The bacteria, which are smaller than the diameter of the dentinal tubules, enter the tubules and destroy the odontoblastic processes that occupy them. The bacteria then travel pulpward in the open tubules and slowly destroy the dentin. Because the bacteria follow the course of the dentinal tubules, a caries lesion that originates around a contact area or in the cervical area of a tooth extends in an apical direction as it approaches the pulp. Notice the direction of the dentinal tubules in Figures 5-1, 5-2, and 5-22.

The horizontal spread of caries is considerably more rapid in dentin than in enamel. A tooth with only a small area of caries visible on the surface may be so extensively carious in the dentin that clinical restoration is impossible. One can easily understand why the tooth shown in Figure 5-21 was lost, but the occlusal surface of this tooth showed too little damage to warn even an observant patient of the probably serious condition inside the tooth.

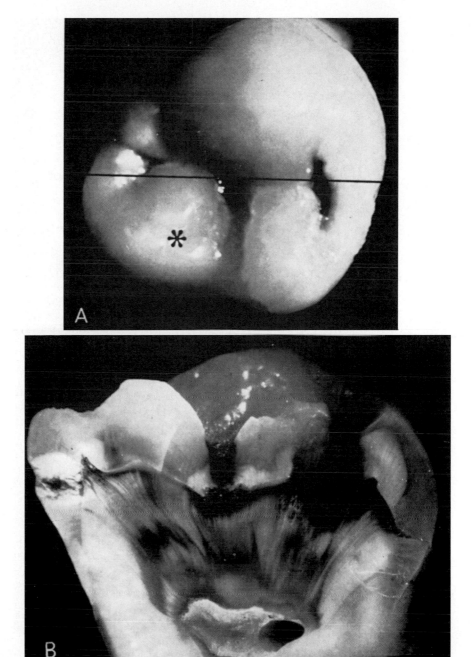

Figure 5–23. A. This maxillary molar shows evidence of caries in the central fossa and mesial triangular fossa, but the casual observer scarcely expects what is revealed when the buccal side of the tooth (asterisk) is ground away. **B.** Caries has penetrated to the pulp cavity and spread laterally, thereby undermining the enamel of the entire occlusal surface. (Notice the curvatures of the dentinal tubules.)

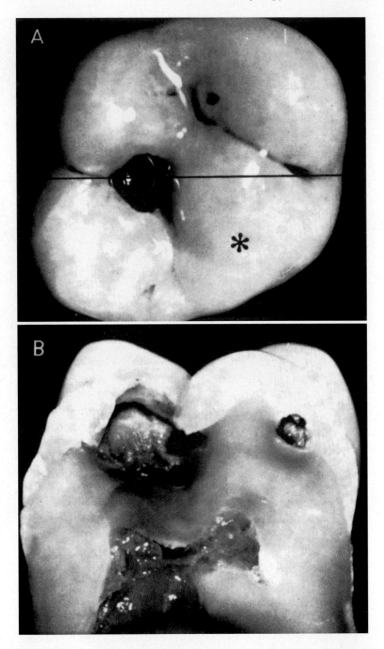

Figure 5–24. A. Caries is obvious in the central fossa of this maxillary molar, and an area of possible caries is seen in the lingual developmental groove. When the mesial surface of the tooth was removed (asterisk), completely unsupported enamel was exposed around the central fossa and suspicious area in the groove. **B.** Notice the extent of caries in the dentin.

The teeth shown in Figures 5-23 and 5-24 had a larger surface area of visible caries, and the enamel around the point of entry was so seriously undermined that a large part of it was unsupported. With this kind of condition, the occlusal enamel often collapses completely when the patient bites on some relatively soft food.

The progress of dental caries through dentin is often retarded, but not stopped, by defense reactions that occur in the pulp. One such reaction is the production of sclerotic dentin. From the pulp tissue, calcium salts are deposited in the dentinal tubules and cause them to become filled with mineral substances. Consequently, the progress of bacterial invasion is slowed. Another defense reaction against caries is the formation of reparative dentin where the bacteria-filled tubules reach the pulp. The resultant increase in the thickness of the dentin wall helps to temporarily protect the tooth pulp against the invasion of the disease. In a tooth from which the pulp has been removed, these defense changes cannot occur.

Another particularly important characteristic of dentin is the location of Tomes' granular layer and its effect on the patient's comfort. As we have seen, Tomes' granular layer consists of a narrow band of unmineralized areas in the root dentin immediately beneath the cementum. In nearly all mouths, natural aging leads to the gradual recession of the gingiva and a resultant exposure of the cementum at the necks of the teeth (see Chapter 11). In performing oral prophylaxis, this exposed cervical cementum must be cleaned. This means working very close to Tomes' granular layer, which is very sensitive because it is unmineralized and in close contact with the odontoblastic processes. Therefore, the patient may experience pain and find this area of exposed cementum sensitive to hot or cold foods. A patient with exposed cervical cementum may believe that he has caries in this area because of pain experienced during eating or while brushing his teeth. Such discomforts are more noticeable when the cervical cementum first becomes exposed. After the cervical cementum has been exposed to the oral environment for several weeks or months, the dentin beneath the exposed surface usually becomes sclerotic (Fig. 5-21), and the patient ceases to notice discomfort.

SUGGESTED READINGS

Brannstrom M, Garberoglio R. The dentinal tubules and the odontoblast processes. A scanning electron microscopic study. Acta Odontol Scand 1972;30:291–311.

Pashley DH. Dynamics of the pulpo-dentin complex. Crit Rev Oral Biol Med 1996;7:104–133.

Scott DB, Simmelink JW, Nygaard V. Structural aspects of dental caries. J Dent Res 1974;53:165–178.

Thomas HF, Payne RC. The ultrastructure of dentinal tubules from erupted human premolar teeth. J Dent Res 1983;65:532–536.

The biology of dentin and pulp. Proceedings of an international workshop. Charlotte, NC, June 10–13, 1984. J Dent Res 1985;64 Spec No:481–633.

6 *Tooth Pulp*

LOCATION

The pulp, located in the interior of the tooth, is enclosed within the dentin, with which it has a close physiologic relationship. It occupies the pulp cavity; more specifically, it fills the pulp chamber in the crown and the root canal in the root and connects with the periodontal ligament at the apical foramen (see Figs. 1-12, 4-1, and 5-2). Anatomically, the outline of a young pulp cavity mirrors the outline of the surface of the tooth (Fig. 6-1).

ORIGIN

The *dental papilla* (mesenchyme) of the *tooth germ* undergoes growth and development and becomes the tooth pulp. Cells of the mesenchymal tissue differentiate into fibroblasts and odontoblasts. The fibroblasts form and maintain the intercellular substance of the pulp, and odontoblasts form the dentin. Blood vessels and nerves that are in the dental papilla remain to supply the pulp tissue.

COMPOSITION

Tooth pulp is the only nonmineralized tissue of a tooth. It is a soft connective tissue and, like other connective tissues, is made of *cells*, *intercellular substance*, and *tissue fluid* (Fig. 6-2). The pulp tissue of older teeth has relatively fewer cells and more intercellular substance than does that of younger teeth.

Although the cells of young pulp tissue are chiefly fibroblasts, specialized cells—histocytes, undifferentiated mesenchymal cells, and odontoblasts—are also present.

The intercellular substance of the pulp consists of the ground substance and the fibrous substance. The ground substance is a jelly-like material in which all the cellular and fibrous elements of the pulp tissue are suspended. The fibrous substance is a meshwork of minute collagen fibrils.

Tooth pulp contains blood vessels and nerves. Many teeth also contain mineralized structures called denticles (pulp stones) and diffuse mineralizations.

COMPONENTS OF THE PULP

Fibroblast cells are more numerous than any other kind of cell in the pulp (Figs. 6-2 and 6-3). They often are described as star-shaped because of the irregular, pointed

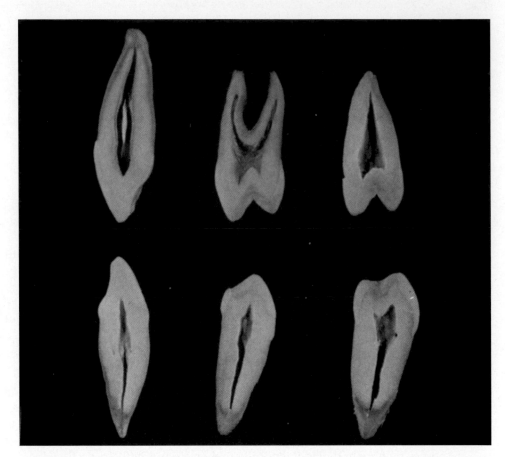

Figure 6–1. These human teeth were ground down in a faciolingual direction to illustrate the anatomic features of the pulp cavity. Notice that the outline of the pulp cavity somewhat mirrors the outer surface of the tooth. From left to right, the maxillary (above) and mandibular (below) teeth shown are the canine, first premolar, and second premolar.

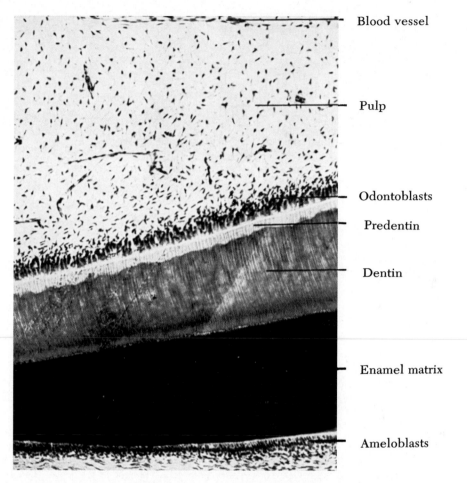

Blood vessel

Pulp

Odontoblasts

Predentin

Dentin

Enamel matrix

Ameloblasts

Figure 6–2. A section through a developing tooth of a pig. The tissues are similar to those of a human tooth. The dark-stained, as yet unmineralized, enamel matrix is covered on its outer surface by the layer of ameloblasts, which are beginning to lose their columnar shape (see Chapter 3). The dentin contains dentinal tubules that extend from the dentinoenamel junction to the pulp. The unmineralized layer of dentin next to the pulp is called predentin or dentinoid and is stained a lighter color than the earlier-formed, mineralized dentin. The pulp cells next to the predentin are the odontoblasts; most of the other cells seen in the pulp are fibroblasts. Nerves and collagen fibers are not seen in this preparation; the latter require a special stain. Small blood vessels are scattered throughout the pulp tissue, and a larger blood vessel is seen at the top.

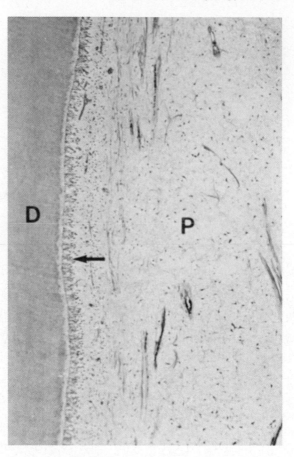

Figure 6–3. Microscopic view of a section cut through an area of pulp (P) and dentin (D). Cell bodies of odontoblasts (arrow) are prominently arranged in a layer along the dentin. The light line between the cell bodies and the darker-stained dentin is the predentin layer. Scattered among the other cells of the pulp are blood vessels and nerves. See Fig. 6-4 for a higher magnification of a similar section.

outlines of their cytoplasm. Fibroblasts are responsible for the formation of the intercellular substance of pulp tissue.

Histocytes and undifferentiated mesenchymal[1] cells are located throughout the pulp near the capillaries. They are part of the defense mechanism of the pulp and respond to pulp injury by changing into the defense cells as seen in any inflammatory reaction.

The *odontoblasts* are specialized connective tissue cells located next to the dentin (Figs. 6-4, 6-5, and 6-6). They are roughly cylindric in shape, somewhat longer than they are wide, and contain an oval-shaped nucleus. They are peculiar cells in that their cytoplasm does not remain entirely in the pulp. The cytoplasm of the odontoblast surrounds the nucleus in the usual manner of cells, but the remainder is stretched out in a long, thin tail that enters a dentinal tubule and extends to the dentinoenamel or the dentinocemental junction (Fig. 6-7, see Fig.

---

[1] Pronounced *měs ěn kǐ mål.*

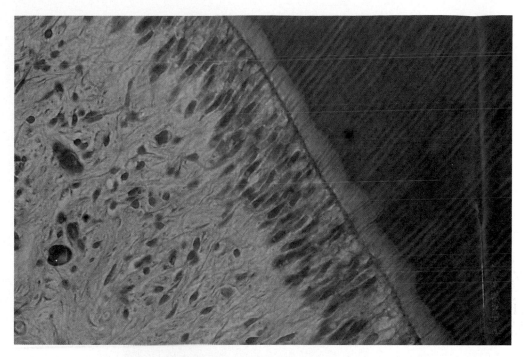

Figure 6–4. (See Color Plates) Higher magnification of an area of pulp and dentin. The prominent cell bodies of the odontoblasts are arranged along the lighter-stained predentin layer. On close inspection, the odontoblast cell processes are seen passing into the dentinal tubules.

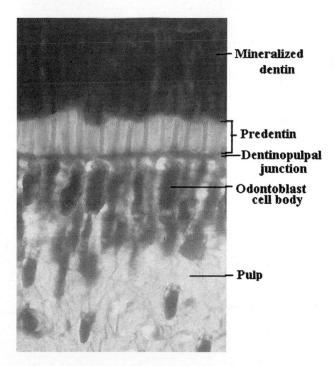

Figure 6–5. High-power magnification of odontoblasts showing their dentinopulpal relation. The cell body and cell processes are located in the pulp and dentin, respectively. Cell processes can be seen passing through the predentin layer (see Fig. 5-10).

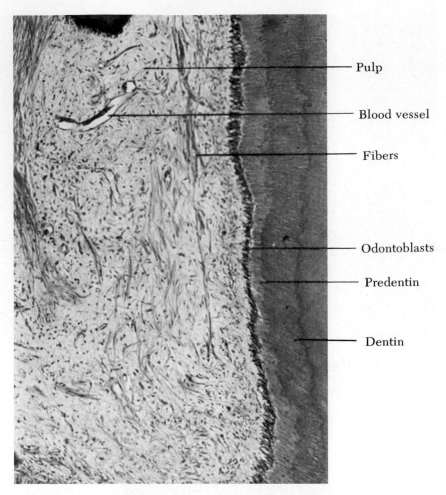

Figure 6–6. Photomicrograph of a section cut through the pulp and dentin of an older tooth. The increase of fibers within the pulp is clearly seen (compare to Figs. 6-3 and 6-4).

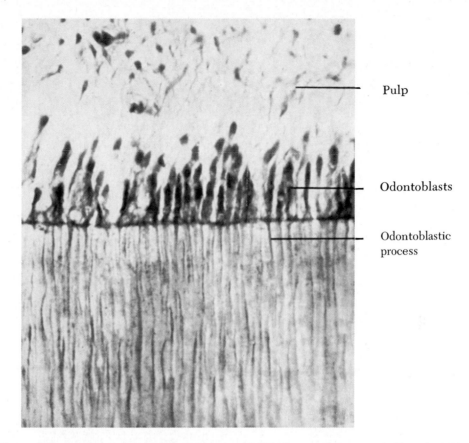

Figure 6–7. A section cut through the pulp and predentin of a young human tooth. The odontoblasts are dark-stained columnar cells. The nuclei and part of the cytoplasm of the odontoblasts are in the pulp; long (odontoblastic) cell processes extend into the dentinal tubules.

5-10). This cytoplasmic tail of the odontoblast is called an *odontoblastic process.* When a process crosses the dentinoenamel junction into the enamel, the portion of the process that is in the enamel is called an enamel spindle (see Figs. 4-20 and 4-21).

Blood vessels are plentiful in young pulp (Figs. 6-8, 6-9, and 6-10). Small branches from the superior or inferior alveolar artery enter the tooth through the apical foramen. As they pass through the root canal to the pulp chamber, they divide into capillaries. The circulating blood is collected into veins that pass out from the pulp through the apical foramen. *Lymphatic vessels* also have been identified in the pulp.

Along the blood vessels, nerves enter the tooth through the apical foramen and provide the pulp with a rich nerve supply (Figs. 6-9 and 6-10). The maxillary teeth are supplied by branches from the second division and the mandibular teeth by branches from the third division of the trigeminal nerve. At the inner ends of the odontoblast cells, the nerves in the pulp form a network, with some nerve fibers having endings on the odontoblasts. This arrangement helps to account for the sensitivity of the dentin, because the odontoblasts have part of their cytoplasm in

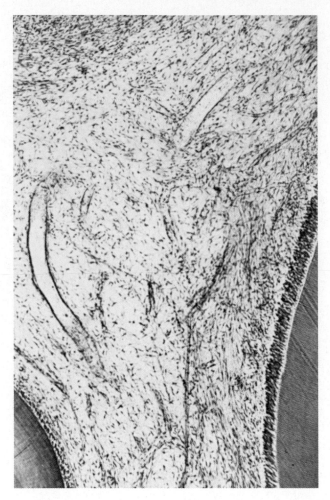

Figure 6–8. Photomicrograph of an area of pulp tissue extending from the wider pulp chamber (above) into the narrower root canal (below). Dentin is seen in the lower left and right sides of the picture. Clearly evident are the many profiles of blood vessels and nerves throughout the pulp.

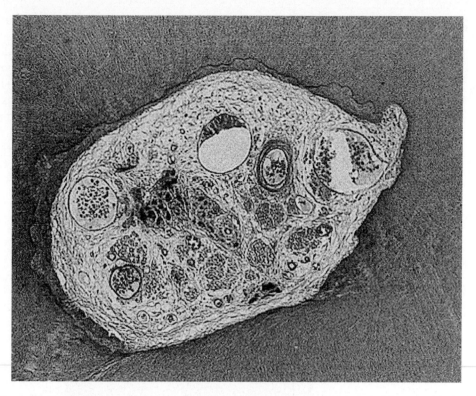

Figure 6–9. Microscopic view of a horizontal section of pulp tissue near the apical foramen. Note the relative size and distribution of blood vessels and nerves in this cross section. See Fig. 6-10 for a high-power view of this site.

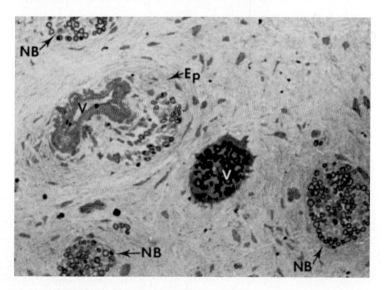

Figure 6–10. Photomicrograph of the center of apical human pulp tissue, cut in cross section. Note thickness of nerve sheath or epineurium (EP) when nerves are associated with blood vessels (V). NB, nerve bundles. (Courtesy Dr. Al Reader, College of Dentistry, Ohio State University.)

the dentinal tubules. Some investigators have seen structures in the dentinal tubules that they have identified as nerves.

Denticles (*pulp stones*) are mineralized bodies of an irregularly rounded shape and frequently are found in the pulp (Figs. 6-11, 6-12, and 6-13). They may lie free in the soft tissue or may be attached to the dentin wall. Denticles vary in shape and size, with size increasing with the age of the tooth. Generally, they are regarded as of little clinical importance, except when they interfere with endodontic treatment. Denticles are never a source of infection.

Diffuse mineralizations are small, thin scatterings of calcified material frequently found in the pulps of older teeth, usually in the root canals (see Figs. 1-14, 5-2, and 6-14). Clinically, they are usually unimportant.

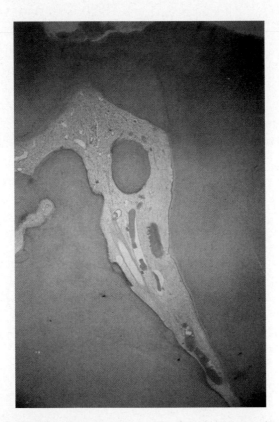

Figure 6–11. (See Color Plates) Longitudinal section of an old human molar. The tissue of the pulp chamber (above) continues into a root canal (below). A large pulp stone (denticle) in the pulp chamber is surrounded by pulp tissue that contains age-related changes (e.g., fewer cells, a deeply stained intercellular substance indicating an alteration of the organic components, possibly an increase of collagen fibrils, and pulpal mineralization). Notice the prominent blood vessels, some of which are engorged with blood cells.

Figure 6–13. (See Color Plates) Photomicrograph of a section through the pulp chamber of an old molar tooth. Pulp stones of different sizes and shapes are visible. A large pulp stone is attached to the pulpal wall of the dentin. Notice the age-related changes in the pulp.

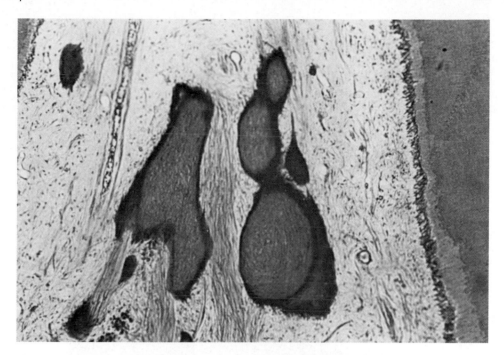

Figure 6–12. Free pulp stones in a normal-appearing pulp tissue of a human molar. The fibers seen between and below the pulp stones are nerves. A blood vessel is conspicuous to the left of the pulp stones. To the right, the odontoblastic layer is in place along the predentin.

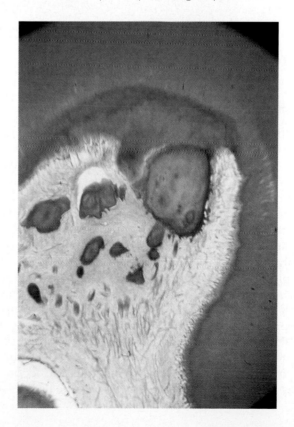

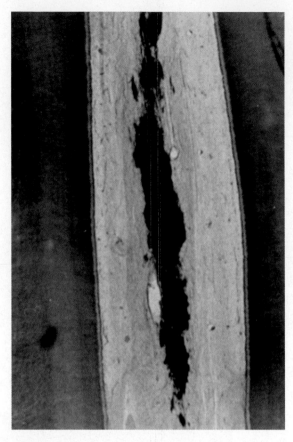

Figure 6–14. Photomicrograph of a portion of a root canal shows diffuse mineralization within the pulp tissue.

ZONES OF THE PULP

Three distinct histologic zones or layers are present in young, healthy pulp and are located at the periphery of the pulp. In a horizontal or cross section of a tooth (Figs. 6-15, 6-16, and 6-17), the zones are seen as circular layers, one within another, around the outer area of the pulp. Each zone is given a descriptive histologic name. The outermost layer, next to the predentin layer of the dentin, is called the *odontoblastic zone* and contains the cell bodies of the odontoblasts. Passing inward toward the pulp core or center is the *cell-free* zone, so named because of its relative lack of cells. Inward from the cell-free zone is the *cell-rich* zone, so called because of its relatively high number of cells (Fig. 6-17).

Physiologically, each pulp zone carries out certain functions. In addition to forming the dentin, the odontoblastic zone most likely also serves as the first line of defense. Because of its prominent position in the pulp, the odontoblastic zone can interpret external stimuli and pass the information to the other cells and nerves of the pulp. The cell-free zone most likely serves as a buffer. Its position between the odontoblastic and cell-rich zones allows room for the cells of these two zones to move freely in and out of the area without obstruction. The innermost, cell-rich zone may be considered a cell reservoir because its cells are capable of differenti-

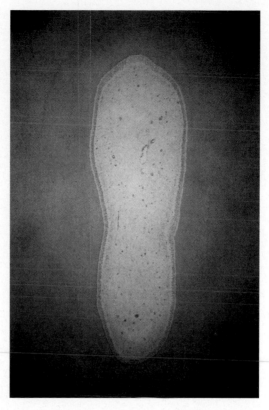

Figure 6–15. (See Color Plates) Horizontal section of a tooth shows a young pulp tissue enclosed within the dentin. From the light-stained predentin toward the center or core of the pulp are the following pulp zones: odontoblastic, cell-free, and cell-rich. See Fig. 6-16 for a clear view of the zones in high magnification.

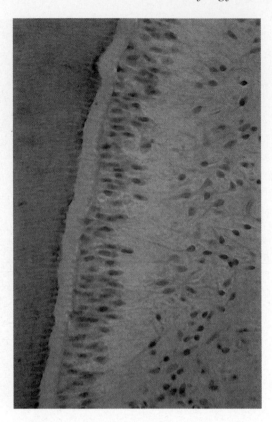

Figure 6–16. (See Color Plates) This high magnification of the pulp and dentin complex clearly delineates the three pulp zones. The odontoblastic zone is made prominent by its position between the light-stained predentin (left) and the light area of the cell-free zone (right). The cell-rich zone is just to the right of the cell-free zone.

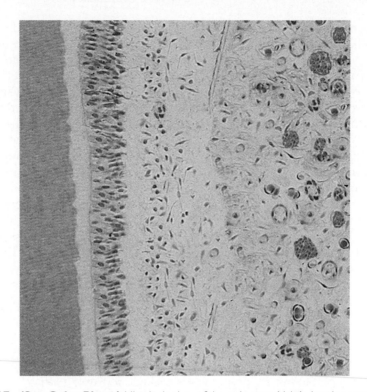

Figure 6–17. (See Color Plates) Histologic view of the pulp core (right) showing cross sections of larger blood vessels and nerves. Note the density of these structures in the core area in relation to the dentopulpal junction at the left. Can you identify the zones or layers of the pulp?

ating into new odontoblasts. If existing odontoblasts degenerate, cells from the cell-rich zone move through the cell-free layer to the degeneration site and differentiate into new odontoblasts. The new odontoblasts form reparative dentin and protect the pulp from the original cause of the degeneration.

An understanding of the normal histologic appearance and position of the three zones is essential for anyone interested in pulp research. Any deviations in the arrangement of the zones, under experimental conditions, should be considered abnormal.

FUNCTIONS OF THE PULP

For purposes of description, the functions of tooth pulp may be described as formative, sensory, nutritive, and defensive.

Formative function. The odontoblasts, the cell bodies (nuclear part) of which lie at the periphery of the pulp, are responsible for the formative function. They produce the collagen fibrils and, while the pulp is young and healthy, the ground substance (organic matrix) of dentin. Naturally, the formative function ceases if the odontoblasts degenerate or if the entire pulp is removed during endodontic therapy.

Sensory function. Tooth pulp is sensitive to external stimuli, and nerves in the pulp are responsible for some of the sensation experienced by an individual when a stimulus is applied to the tooth. The sensation educed by stimuli received by a tooth pulp is a sensation of pain. A person cannot differentiate between extremes of heat (hot coffee) and of cold (ice cream) applied to the tooth. Slight pressures on a tooth, however, produce a sensation of pressure or touch. Most of this sensation is caused by pressure on the periodontal ligament.

Nutritive function. Tooth pulp is a living tissue with a blood supply and receives nutrients from the bloodstream. Nutrients most likely enter the dentinal tubules through the odontoblastic processes or around the outside of the odontoblastic process and may be carried as far as the dentinoenamel and dentinocemental junctions.

Because of the necessary brevity of this discussion, one should realize that the nutritive function of the pulp and the general nutrition of the individual cannot be associated with the presence or absence of dental caries. Dental caries is a disease that begins on the outside surface of the tooth and is a process of an entirely different nature.

Defensive function. Defense reactions of the pulp are expressed in several ways. Pulp may display an inflammatory reaction, change the character of existing dentin (sclerosis), or produce additional dentin (reparative dentin).

Damaged pulp displays an inflammatory reaction, and cells common to any site of inflammation appear. Some of these defense cells are derived from histiocytes and undifferentiated mesenchymal cells of the pulp; some are carried into the pulp by the bloodstream from their points of origin in the bone marrow and lymph nodes. As the defense cells become effective in controlling the damaging process, the pulp may produce sclerosis of the existing dentin and may lay down reparative dentin along the pulpal wall (see Figs. 5-18 and 5-19).

Sclerosis of the dentin involves the filling in of the dentinal tubules, usually in a restricted area, with calcium salts. Consequently, dentin in this area is a solid mineralized tissue instead of a tissue perforated with tubules that contain odontoblastic processes (see Figs. 5-1 and 5-2). Sclerotic dentin usually occurs beneath a caries lesion, and its presence tends to retard the progress of the destruction of tooth tissue. The stimulus to the pulp that causes dentin sclerosis is received through the dentinal tubules.

On the inner or pulpal surface of the sclerotic dentin, odontoblasts of the pulp may produce varying amounts of *reparative dentin* as a defense reaction and provide the pulp with additional protection against external irritation. The formation of reparative and sclerotic dentin occurs in aging teeth (in which infection is not a factor) as a result of the stimulation produced by attrition (see Fig. 5-22).

The saying "A chain is only as strong as its weakest link" may be applied to the functions of the pulp. Consider each function as an interlocking link in a chain. When any link is altered, the others are weakened, and a break in the chain of function occurs. If an individual receives a severe blow to a tooth from an outside source and the tooth is displaced, the blood vessels entering the apical foramen could be severed. Such damage to the blood supply to the pulp would result in loss of nutritive function and weakening of other functions; complete degeneration of pulp tissue would follow.

AGE-RELATED CHANGES IN THE PULP

Just as age brings about changes in other parts of the body, the changes it brings about in the pulps of teeth are universal and normal and should not be regarded as pathologic. The continued formation of reparative dentin with increasing age causes the pulp chamber to become smaller and the root canals to become narrower. In some old teeth that show heavy attrition or long-standing dental caries, the pulp chamber may be entirely filled by reparative dentin. The cells of the pulp which are numerous in young teeth decrease with age, and the fibrous intercellular substance is relatively increased (Figs. 6-11 and 6-13). Old tooth pulps are composed mostly of fibrous intercellular substance, and blood and nerve supplies decrease with age. Denticles are larger and more numerous in old teeth, and diffuse mineralizations are increased. However, these changes of the pulp do not alter tooth function.

CLINICAL IMPORTANCE OF THE PULP

A fully developed tooth may function for many years after its pulp has been removed and its pulp canal has been filled. Although the enamel of the tooth becomes more brittle, its function is not affected by the loss of the pulp. The cementum is not affected, nor is the process of continued cementum formation. A tooth without a pulp cannot, however, produce reparative dentin or sclerotic dentin. Loss of a tooth pulp usually results from caries or tooth fracture, with accompanying pulp infection. Careful treatment by the dentist is essential in either case to prevent the infection from traveling through the root canal and apical foramen into the tissues surrounding the tooth, which may result in tooth loss.

SUGGESTED READINGS

Byers MR, Narhi MVO. Dental injury models: experimental tools for understanding neuroinflammatory interactions and polymodal nociceptor functions. Crit Rev Oral Biol Med 1999;10:4–39.

Cohen S, Burns RC, eds. Pathways of the Pulp. 5th Ed. St. Louis: Mosby–Year Book, 1991.

Inoki R, Kudo T, Olgart LM, eds. Dynamic Aspects of the Dental Pulp: Molecular biology, pharmacology, and pathophysiology. New York: Chapman and Hall, 1990.

Olgart L. Neural control of pulpal blood flow. Crit Rev Oral Biol Med 1996;7:159–171.

Shimono M, Maida T, Suda H, and Takahashi K, eds. Dentin/pulpal complex. Tokyo: Quintessence Publishing Co., 1996.

7   Cementum

LOCATION

Cementum is the layer of mineralized tissue that covers the surface of the root of a tooth (Figs. 4-1 and 7-1). It overlies and is attached to the root dentin. Around the cervical part of the root, cementum is approximately 0.05 mm thick; on the apical part of the root of a functioning tooth, it is usually considerably thicker. In the area of the cementoenamel junction, the cementum may have one of three relationships with the enamel of the tooth crown (Fig. 7-2). It may exactly meet the enamel; it may not quite meet the enamel, leaving some dentin exposed; or it may slightly overlap the enamel (Figs. 7-2, 7-3, 7-4, 7-5, and 7-6). This last arrangement is the most common.

Cementogenesis is the name given to the origin and formation of cementum. Review the section on root formation in Chapter 3.

FUNCTIONS OF CEMENTUM

Cementum is not only recognized as a tissue of a tooth, but is also included as a tissue of the periodontium along with the bone of the socket, the periodontal ligament, and the connective tissue of the gingiva. As part of the periodontium, cementum serves its primary function of providing the medium by which the other parts of the periodontium are attached to the tooth. Without cementum, the tooth would not be retained in the socket.

By its anatomic position over the root, cementum protects the underlying dentin, which is subject to resorption if the more resistant cementum is lost. Cementum also serves as a mending tissue at the site of a root fracture. Cementoblasts from the periodontal ligament move into the fracture site and form cementum, thereby uniting the fractured parts.

Physiologically, teeth are subject to attrition (see Figs. 5-20 and 5-21) at their occlusal surfaces. To compensate for this loss of occlusal tissue, cementum is formed at apical and furcation areas of roots. Consequently, cementum is usually thickest at these sites (Fig. 7-1).

In summary, cementum serves as the tooth attachment medium, protects root dentin, serves as the mending tissue in fracture sites, and compensates for loss of tooth tissues at the occlusal surface.

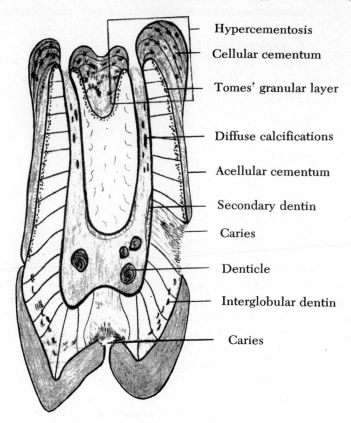

Hypercementosis

Cellular cementum

Tomes' granular layer

Diffuse calcifications

Acellular cementum

Secondary dentin

Caries

Denticle

Interglobular dentin

Caries

Figure 7–1. Drawing of a longitudinal faciolingual section of a maxillary first premolar. The tip of the lingual root shows a large amount of cementum, which is sometimes referred to as hypercementosis. For a photomicrograph of such thick cementum, see Fig. 7-12.

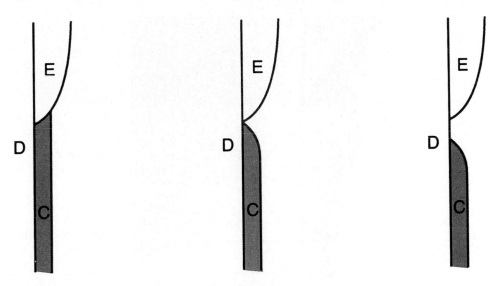

Figure 7–2. Diagrams of the relation of cementum (C) to enamel (E) at the dentinoenamel junction. The most common relation is illustrated at the left, where cementum overlaps the enamel. Illustrated in the center is the next most common relation, where cementum just meets the enamel. The least common relation is illustrated at the right, where cementum does not meet the enamel. Cervical dentin (D) is void of cementum and exposed to the environment.

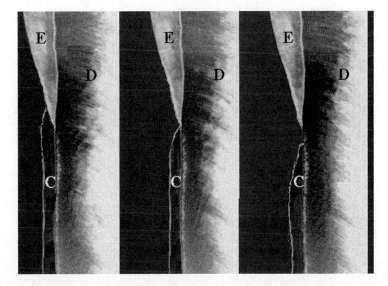

Figure 7–3. Ground sections of teeth showing the relation of cementum to enamel. The most common relationship is at the left, least common at the right (see Fig. 7-2).

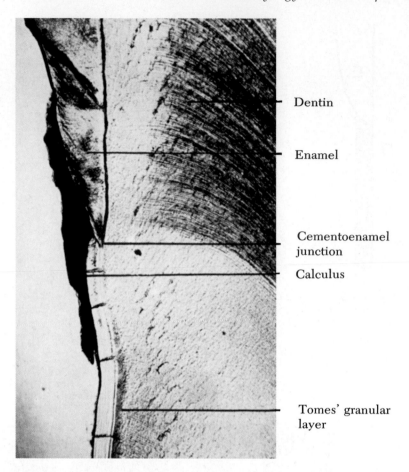

Figure 7–4. Photomicrograph (low power) of a ground section of a tooth in the area of the cementoenamel junction. The cementum slightly overlaps the enamel. Calculus adheres to both enamel and cementum. The four conspicuous lines in the cementum are cracks produced by the grinding of the section. Tomes' granular layer lies beneath the cementum in the dentin. Deeper in the dentin in both the root and crown are irregular dark areas of interglobular dentin. The dentinal tubules are distinct. The darkness of the tubules in the upper right is caused by air that entered the tubules during section preparation; it is not evidence of structural change.

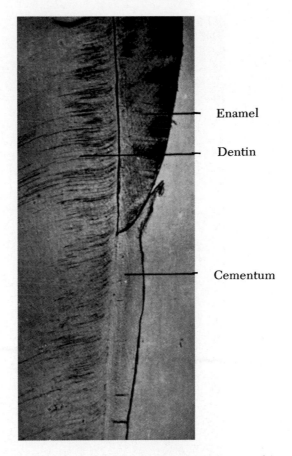

Enamel

Dentin

Cementum

Figure 7–5. Photomicrograph of a ground section of a tooth in the area of the cementoenamel junction. The cementum overlaps the enamel considerably. The separation of cementum from enamel at the border of the cementum is an artifact most likely caused by the drying of the specimen during section preparation; in life, the cementum was most likely fixed firmly against the enamel surface.

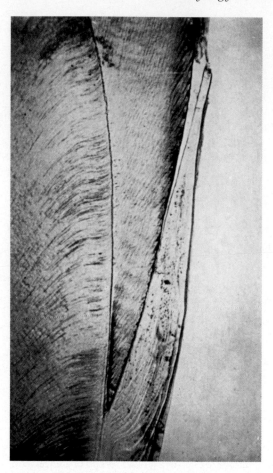

Figure 7–6. Photomicrograph of a ground section of a tooth in the area of the cementoenamel junction. The cementum on this tooth overlaps the enamel to an unusual extent; not many teeth show this amount of overlapping. The separation of cementum from enamel is most likely caused by the drying of the specimen during the preparation. In life, the cementum undoubtedly was firm against the enamel. This is the mesial side of a mandibular molar.

COMPOSITION

Like enamel, dentin, and bone, cementum is made of an organic matrix that contains crystallized mineral substances. Cementum is not as hard as dentin, being about 50% inorganic (mineral) material and about 50% organic substance and water; it has about the same hardness as bone. Cementum may contain cells called *cementocytes* irregularly scattered through it, but it does not contain blood vessels or nerves.

STRUCTURE OF CEMENTUM

The structure of cementum is both similar to and different from that of dentin (see Table 9-1). As in dentin, the organic matrix is composed of a framework of fine collagen fibrils held together by a ground substance that becomes mineralized. Cementum may contain whole cells, whereas dentin contains only processes of pulp cells. Like the other three mineralized tissues of the body, cementum is formed in layers that result in the appositional growth lines seen in histologic sections (Figs. 7-7 and 7-8). These lines are parallel to the long axis of the root. The oldest layer of cementum is next to the root dentin, and the most recent layer is always next to the periodontal ligament.

Histologically, two types of cementum may be seen around a tooth. One type is without cells and called *acellular cementum* (Figs. 7-1, 7-7, 7-8, and 7-9); the other type contains cells and is called *cellular cementum* (Figs. 7-1, 7-8, 7-9, and 7-10).

The organic matrix of both types of cementum is produced by *cementoblasts*, which are located in the periodontal ligament next to the cementum. More specifically, they lie next to the *cementoid layer* (Fig. 7-7), which is the most recent organic matrix formed by the cementoblasts.

The cementoblasts may become surrounded by the organic matrix and, thus, may be converted into cells of the cementum (cementocytes). Cementocytes are connected with one another by the numerous thread-like projections of their cytoplasm. The space in the cementum occupied by the body of the cementocyte is

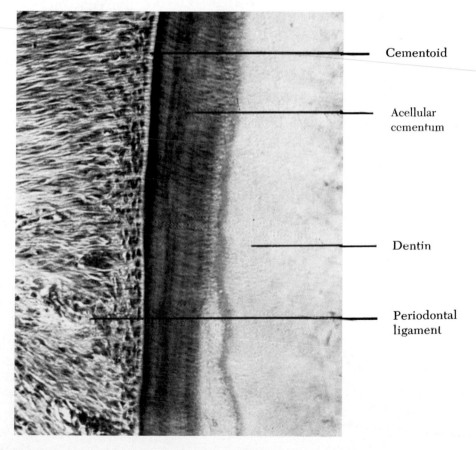

Cementoid

Acellular cementum

Dentin

Periodontal ligament

Figure 7–7. Higher magnification of a section of acellular cementum and adjacent tissues. Clearly seen is the thin cementoid layer, which appears light because it is less mineralized than the rest of the cementum. Cementoblasts are seen along the surface of the cementoid layer within the periodontal ligament. Notice the dark growth lines of the cementum aligned parallel to the surface.

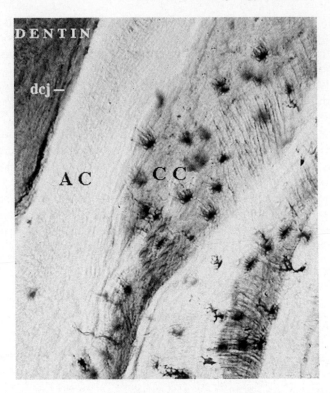

Figure 7–8. (See Color Plates) Ground section of a root area showing acellular cementum (AC) next to the dentinocemental junction (DCJ) and cellular cementum (CC).

Figure 7–10. High power magnification of two cementum lacunae and their radiating canaliculi. The cell body of the cementocyte, which is usually located in the lacuna, and its processes, which occupy the canaliculi, are not seen; they were lost during tissue preparation.

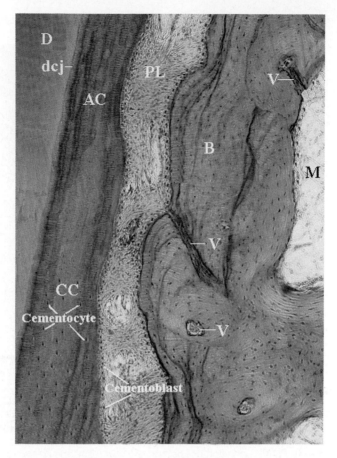

Figure 7–9. (See Color Plates) Demineralized section of an area of acellular cementum (AC) and cellular cementum (CC). D, dentin; PL, periodontal ligament; B, alveolar bone; DCJ, dentinocemental junction; V, vascular canals; M, bone marrow.

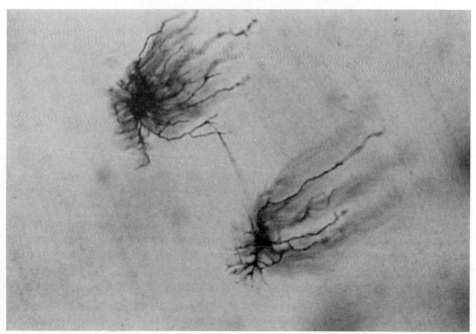

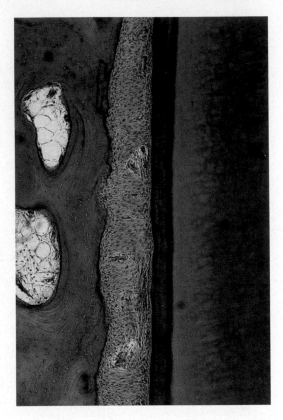

Figure 7–11. Photomicrograph of a portion of a root (right) and adjacent tissues. The darkest-stained tissue is acellular cementum. The bone of the tooth socket (left) encloses two open, clear areas of bone marrow. Between the mineralized cementum and bone is the soft tissue of the periodontal ligament with its many cells. To the right of the dark-stained cementum is dentin.

called a *lacuna* (little space), and the spaces occupied by the cytoplasmic projections of the cementocyte are called *canaliculi* (little canals). Canaliculi of adjacent lacunae may join and connect neighboring lacunae. In cementum, most of the canaliculi are directed toward the periodontal ligament (Figs. 7-10, 7-11, and 7-12).

Ordinarily, cementocytes are not found throughout the entire cementum on the tooth root, and usually the thin cementum on the cervical portion of the root has no cementocytes (Figs. 7-1, 7-4, 7-5, and 7-7). In the apical portion of the root, the cementum is usually relatively thick, and whereas in this region the cementum close to the dentin may have a few cementocytes, the outer layers often contain many irregularly distributed cementocytes (Figs. 7-1, 7-8, 7-9, and 7-12).

Visible in the cementum by microscopic examination are *Sharpey's fibers* (Figs. 7-13, 7-14, 7-15, and 7-16). These ends of the periodontal ligament's bundled fibers have become embedded in the cementum during its formation and attach the periodontal ligament firmly to the tooth (see Chapter 8).

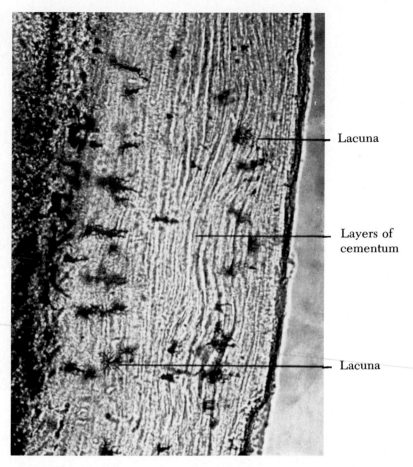

Lacuna

Layers of cementum

Lacuna

Figure 7–12. Photomicrograph of an area of cementum seen with a higher-power objective than that used for Fig. 7-9. Notice the canaliculi leading from the lacunae; they often are directed chiefly toward the outside surface of the root (to the right). The layer-upon-layer formation of cementum is clear. See Fig. 7-7 for a higher magnification of lacunae and their radiating canaliculi.

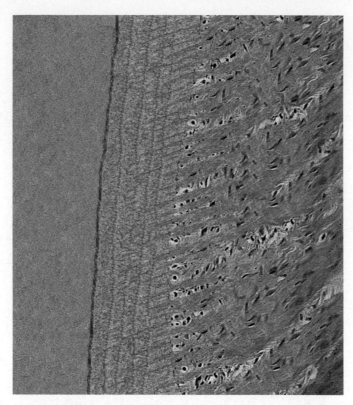

Figure 7–13. (See Color Plates) Histologic view of root (left) and periodontal ligament (right). Ends of collagen fibers of the periodontal ligament are seen passing into acellular cementum where they are identified as Sharpey's fibers. Note the incremental growth lines running longitudinally within the ce-mentum. The dark-stained line is the dentinocemental junction.

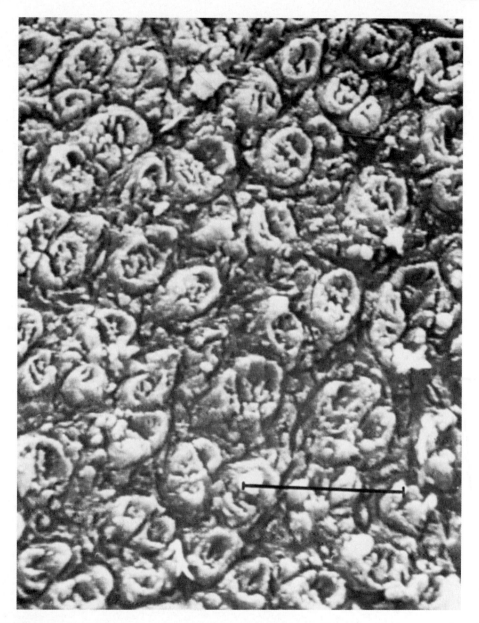

Figure 7–14. Scanning electron micrograph of acellular cementum. The many elevations are points of attachment of Sharpey's fibers. The length of the marker represents 20 microns. (Courtesy Dr. Dennis Foreman, College of Dentistry, Ohio State University.)

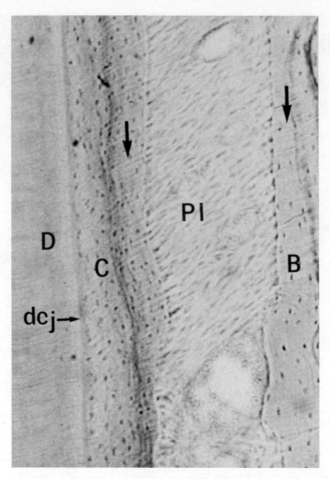

Figure 7–15. Photomicrograph of a section of a root and adjacent tissues. Ends of periodontal ligament (PL) fibers pass into cellular cementum (C) and bone (B) of the tooth socket, consequently becoming the embedded Sharpey's fibers (arrows). D, dentin; DCJ, dentinocemental junction.

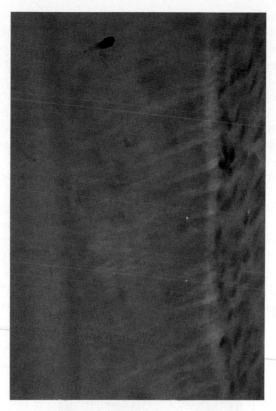

Figure 7–16. (See Color Plates) Higher magnification of a cellular cementum section with clearly visible Sharpey's fibers. Notice the cementoblast within the periodontal ligament arranged along the lighter-stained cementoid layer and the cementocytes within the cementum.

CLINICAL IMPORTANCE OF CEMENTUM

The cementum is part of the mechanism by which a tooth is attached in the tooth socket. Just as the periodontal ligament is attached to the tooth by Sharpey's fibers embedded in the cementum, it is similarly attached to the tooth socket by Sharpey's fibers embedded in the bone (Figs. 7-16 and 8-6). Because of this double attachment, the tooth is literally suspended in its socket.

Cementum most likely continues to be produced intermittently throughout the life of the tooth by cementoblasts of the periodontal ligament. Additions of cementum at the root apex compensate for the loss of crown length, which results from attrition during years of use.

Cementum also repairs damage to the tooth root by replacing lost areas of tooth root that have been resorbed following injury. Although normal vertical pressures or light lateral pressures do not result in damage to the tooth root, severe lateral pressure on a tooth may result not only in resorption of some areas of the bone of the tooth socket, but also in localized resorption of the tooth root. In some cases, underlying dentin and cementum may also be resorbed. When the cause of the resorption is removed before the damage becomes too extensive, new cementum may be laid down over the damaged area, thereby replacing both the lost cementum and the lost dentin.

The presence of *cementoid* (Figs. 7-7 and 7-16) on the outer surface of the root is an important factor in the clinical success of orthodontic treatment. Because cementoid is only slightly mineralized, it undergoes resorption less readily than does bone. When the orthodontist establishes continued light lateral pressure on a tooth by the use of orthodontic appliances, the pressure is transmitted to the periodontal ligament and bone of the tooth socket; the bone, but not the tooth root, is then resorbed. On the opposite side of the tooth socket, where the periodontal ligament is under tension because of this lateral movement, addition of bone takes place, and an actual change occurs in the location of the tooth socket and the position of the tooth (see Chapter 9). The difference between the pressure used by the orthodontist and the pressure that causes damage to the tooth root lies chiefly in the severity of the pressure.

Cementum is sometimes formed in excessive amounts and is called *hypercementosis*, *excementosis*, or *cementum hyperplasia*. It may occur on all or only a few teeth in any mouth, over the entire tooth root or only in localized areas (Fig. 7-1). The causes of excessive cementum formation are not fully known. A large amount of cementum sometimes is useful because it may furnish additional attachment for periodontal ligament fibers, but it may also be a handicap. If excessive cementum occurs as a spicule protruding from the side of the root and interlocking in a re-

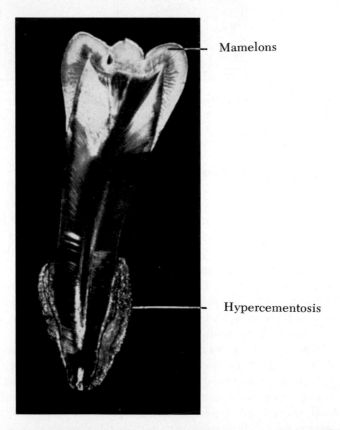

Mamelons

Hypercementosis

Figure 7–17. Photomicrograph (low power) of a ground section of a mandibular incisor, cut mesiodistally. Before this tooth was cut, the apical half of the root resembled a round ball on the end of the tooth (referred to as hypercementosis). Notice the conspicuous mamelons and the pit between the left and center mamelon.

sorbed area of the lamina dura (i.e., the bone of the tooth socket), or if it occurs as excessive cementum at the root apex and produces a ball-shaped root end (Fig. 7-16), extraction of the tooth may be a problem.

Small bodies of cementum called *cementicles* are sometimes found in the periodontal ligament (see Fig. 8-18) and are usually regarded as of no clinical importance.

Like the surfaces of enamel and dentin, the external surface of cementum is susceptible to caries. If the gingiva migrates apically until the cementum becomes exposed to the oral environment, the surface of the cementum is subject to the same caries activity that occurs at the surface of enamel.

SUGGESTED READING

Bosshardt DD, Selvig KA. Dental cementum: the dynamic tissue covering of the root. Periodontology 2000 1997;13:41–75.

MacNeil RL, Somerman MJ. Development and regeneration of the periodontium: parallels and contrast. Periodontology 2000 1999;19:8–20.

8   *Periodontal Ligament*

LOCATION

The periodontal ligament (peri = around; odontos = tooth) is a layer of connective tissue usually less than 0.25 mm in width that surrounds the root of a tooth, occupying the space between the cementum and bone of the tooth socket (Figs. 8-1, 8-2, and 8-3). Because of its position and fibrous makeup, the periodontal ligament is the main suspensory tissue of the periodontium, which includes the cementum of the tooth, the bone of the tooth socket, and the soft connective tissue of the gingiva (Fig. 8-4).

STRUCTURE OF THE PERIODONTAL LIGAMENT

The periodontal ligament is made of cells, ground and fibrous types of intercellular substance, and tissue fluid. The most outstanding constituent is the fibrous intercellular substance that forms the *fibers of the periodontal ligament*, or the protein *collagen*. These fibers are physically constructed to withstand heavy forces, such as those that occur during mastication. Among these fibers are located *fibroblast cells*, *blood vessels*, and *nerves* (Fig. 8-3); in some areas, small groups or strings of epithelial cells and *cementicles* are also found. In addition to these components, specialized cells often function during cementum (cementoblasts) and bone (osteoblasts) formation (Fig. 8-5); other specialized cells are associated with the resorption of cementum (cementoclasts) and bone (osteoclasts). Undifferentiated mesenchymal cells, macrophages, and blood-borne cells (such as lymphocytes) are also present.

The width of the periodontal ligament ranges from 0.12 to 0.33 mm (Figs. 8-4 and 8-6) and varies around different teeth and in different areas around the same tooth. Decreased function of the tooth appears to be accompanied by decreased width of the periodontal ligament.

Bundles of periodontal ligament fibers are attached to the cementum that covers the tooth root and to the bone of the tooth socket on either side of the ligament. When the cementum and bone are forming, ends of bundles of the periodontal ligament fibers become entrapped in the forming hard tissue. This attachment serves to hold the tooth firmly in the jaw, and the entrapped heavy collagen fiber bundles of the periodontal ligament are referred to collectively as *Sharpey's fibers* (Figs. 8-7 and 8-8). The only exceptions are fibers around the cervix of the tooth that attach to either the gingiva or the adjacent tooth (Figs. 8-1 and Fig 8-9).

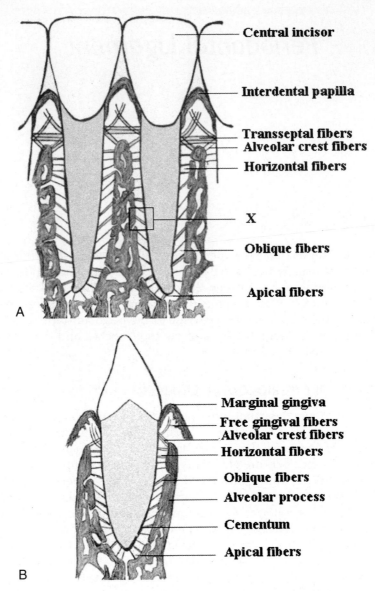

Figure 8–1. Diagrammatic illustration of the arrangement of periodontal ligament fibers around the tooth roots of mandibular incisors. The width of the periodontal ligament is exaggerated to show the direction of the fibers. **A.** Facial view. **B.** Proximal view. Area X in Fig. 8-1A is shown in histologic detail in Figs. 8-2 and 8-3.

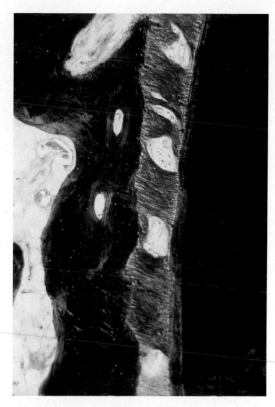

Figure 8–2. (See Color Plates) Histologic section of an area comparable in position to area X in Fig. 8-1A. It was specifically prepared to reveal the arrangement of the collagen fibers of the periodontal ligament between the bone of the socket (left) and the cementum (right). The open areas among the collagen fibers of the periodontal ligament are sites for blood vessels and nerves; the open areas in the bone are sites of bone marrow. Cells were eliminated from the tissues during histologic preparation. See Fig. 8-3 for cellular detail.

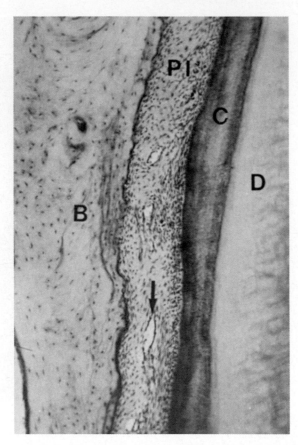

Figure 8–3. Microscopic view of an area similar to Fig. 8-2 and area X in Fig. 8-1A. Notice the relation of the highly cellular periodontal ligament (PL) to the acellular cementum (C) and to the cellular bone of the tooth socket (B). At this magnification, the numerous cells of the periodontal ligament and bone appear as small dots. The open spaces in the periodontal ligament are blood vessels (arrow). Collagen fibers of the periodontal ligament, although present, are not clearly seen in this preparation. D, dentin.

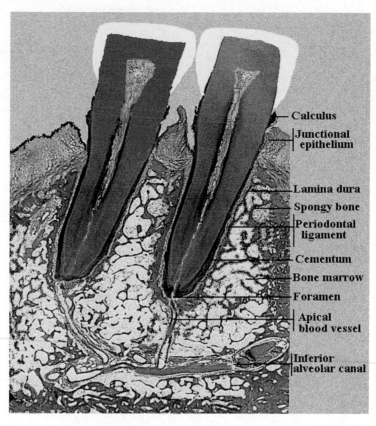

Calculus

Junctional
epithelium

Lamina dura

Spongy bone

Periodontal
ligament

Cementum

Bone marrow

Foramen

Apical
blood vessel

Inferior
alveolar canal

Figure 8–4. Mesiodistal section through the mandibular central incisors. Note the position and width of the periodontal ligament at different sites.

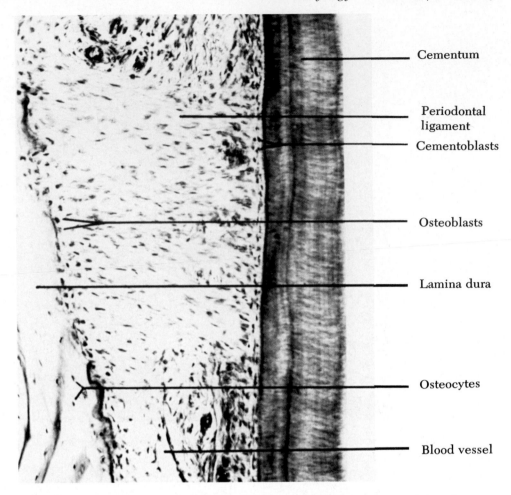

Cementum

Periodontal ligament

Cementoblasts

Osteoblasts

Lamina dura

Osteocytes

Blood vessel

Figure 8–5. Photomicrograph of a section of a human periodontal ligament and the adjacent cementum and lamina dura. Cementoblasts are seen along the surface of the cementoid layer of the cementum. Osteoblasts are clearly seen along the surface of the lamina dura (wall of tooth socket). These cells are specialized connective tissue cells. The majority of cells seen scattered throughout the periodontal ligament are fibroblasts. They are located along the principal fiber bundles, which appear white in this photo.

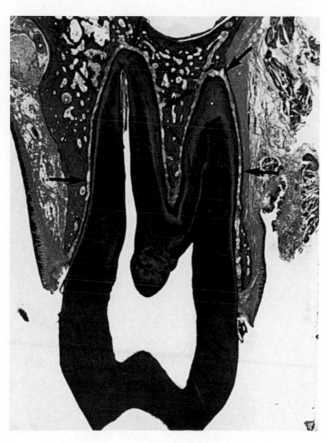

Figure 8–6. Faciolingual section through a maxillary first premolar and its surrounding tissues. Notice the narrow width of the periodontal ligament (arrows) around the roots. The open area above the root apices is the maxillary sinus. Pulp tissue and enamel were lost during histologic processing.

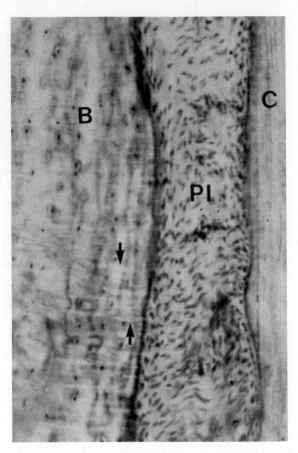

Figure 8–7. Photomicrograph showing the relation of the periodontal ligament (PL) to the cementum (C) and bone of the socket (B). Of particular interest are the Sharpey's fibers embedded in the bone, which appear as white horizontal lines (arrows) in this photo.

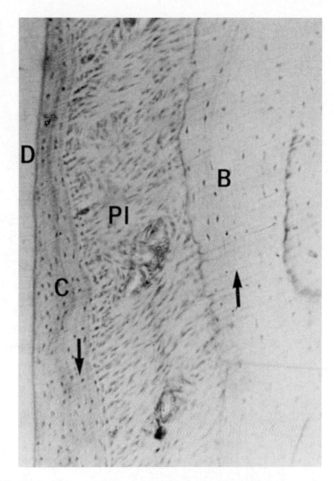

Figure 8–8. Histologic section of the periodontal ligament (PL) and its surrounding structures. Here, the ends of the collagen fiber bundles of the periodontal ligament are seen both in cementum (C) and bone (B). In both cementum and bone, these embedded ends are called Sharpey's fibers (arrows). D, dentin.

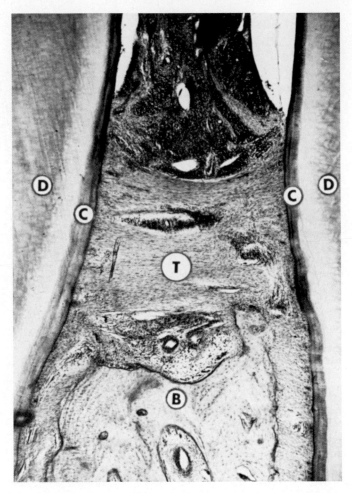

Figure 8–9. Microscopic view of the interdental area between the lower permanent lateral and central incisors. Transseptal fibers (T) pass from the mesial cementum (C) of the lateral incisor (left), over the interdental bone (B), to the distal cementum (C) of the central incisor. The area above the transseptal fibers is the interdental papilla of the gingiva. D, dentin. For diagrammatic comparison, see Fig. 8-1.

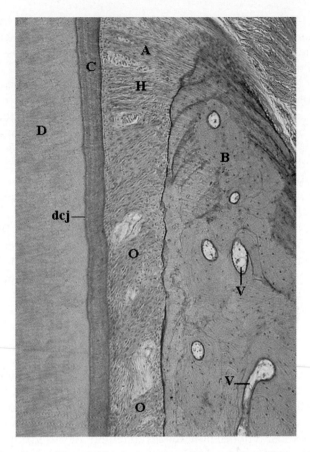

Figure 8–10. (See Color Plates) Histologic section of the periodontal ligament showing position, direction, and relation of alveolar crest fibers (A), horizontal fibers (H), and oblique fibers (O). C, cementum; D, dentin; DCJ, dentinocemental junction; B, bone (alveolar); V, vascular canals of bone.

Although large bundles of fibers are attached to both cementum and bone, each fiber of each bundle does not necessarily extend uninterrupted from cementum to bone. Some individual fibers may extend from cementum or from bone toward the center of the periodontal ligament, where they may terminate and their ends may be interwoven with ends of fibers from the opposite direction.

Around a nonfunctioning tooth (a tooth that is not in occlusion with the teeth in the opposing arch) the periodontal ligament fibers are relaxed and wavy, with no definite orientation (Fig. 9-13). However, around a tooth that is in firm function, the fiber bundles are stretched straight and have characteristic orientations on different areas of the tooth root (Figs. 8-1, 8-8, and 8-10). These large, well-oriented bundles of fibers are referred to as the *principal fibers of the periodontal ligament*.

PRINCIPAL FIBERS OF THE PERIODONTAL LIGAMENT

The principal fibers of the periodontal ligament that surround a heavily functioning tooth have such a clear and consistent arrangement that they have been classified into seven groups. Each group is named according to its location and orientation: (1) the free gingival fibers, (2) the transseptal fibers, (3) the alveolar crest fibers, (4) the horizontal fibers, (5) the oblique fibers, (6) the apical fibers, and (7) the interradicular fibers (inter = between or among; radicular = root). Study the position of these groups of fibers in Figures 8-1 and 8-5 as you read their description in the text.

Free gingival fibers are located around the cervical part of the root. Bundles of these fibers are embedded at one end in the cementum and extend from the cementum into the gingiva that surrounds the neck of the tooth. In the gingiva, the heavy bundles of fibers separate into individual fibers and intermingle with the connective tissue fibers of the gingiva. Examine Figures 8-1 and 11-7 for the location and arrangement of the free gingival fibers. Notice that a pressure applied on the incisal (or occlusal) part of the tooth causes the free gingival fibers to be stretched taut; consequently, this group of fibers functions to hold the gingiva firmly to the tooth surface.

Transseptal fibers are located just apical of the gingival fiber group, only on the mesial and distal sides of the tooth. Bundles of these fibers are embedded at one end in the cementum of one tooth and at the other end in the cementum of an adjacent tooth. With the exception of the maxillary and mandibular central incisors, where the mesial sides of the right and left teeth are connected by these fibers, the transseptal fibers extend from the cementum on the mesial side of one tooth to the cementum on the distal side of an adjacent tooth. Notice in Figures 8-1 and 8-9 how they cross over the top of the bone between the teeth. These fibers help to ensure that the teeth remain in proper relationship to one another.

Alveolar crest fibers are located at the level of the alveolar crest (the margin of the bone that surrounds the tooth root). These fiber bundles are embedded on either side of the periodontal ligament in the cementum of the tooth root and in the alveolar crest. Alveolar crest fibers are found all around the tooth. Examine Figures 8-1 and 8-10, and notice how the arrangement of this group of fibers helps to resist horizontal movements of the tooth.

Horizontal fibers are located apical of the alveolar crest fibers and are embedded in the cementum of the tooth root and in the bone of the tooth socket. They lie in a horizontal position relative to the jaw bone and also are found all around the tooth root. Examine the arrangement of these fibers in Figures 8-1 and 8-10 to see how they function to resist horizontal pressures applied to the tooth crown.

Oblique fibers are located immediately apical of the horizontal group. They are attached to the cementum and bone of the tooth socket, and they run in an oblique, or diagonal, direction. Look at the orientation of these fibers in Figures 8-1, 8-11, and 8-13. The end attached to the bone is always located more toward the tooth crown than is the end attached to the cementum. Imagine a pressure applied vertically to the incisal (or occlusal) surface of the tooth. Such a pressure stretches the oblique fibers taut, and the tooth is literally suspended in its socket. The result of such vertical pressure is a pull on, rather than a pressure on, both the cementum of the tooth root and the bone of the alveolus (tooth socket). This pull or tension is fortunate, because continued pressure on bone ordinarily results in bone resorption. This group of strong oblique fiber bundles prevents the apex of the root from being jammed against the bottom of the socket.

At the transition between the oblique fibers and the radiating apical fibers is a small region in which the fibers again extend in a horizontal plane. Although these

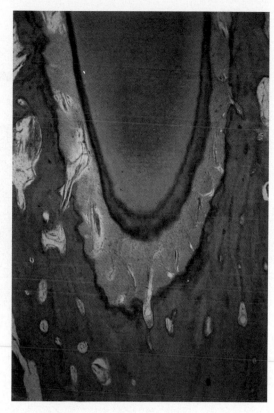

Figure 8–11. (See Color Plates) Histologic view of the apical part of a tooth, the apical fibers of the periodontal ligament, and the surrounding alveolar bone. Compare the arrangement of the apical fibers shown here to those illustrated in Figs. 8-1 and 8-13.

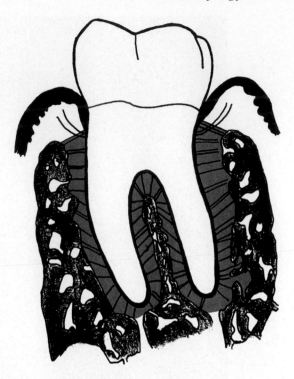

Figure 8–12. Mesiodistal view of a lower permanent first molar and periodontium. The arrangement of the periodontal ligament fibers in association with the tooth and surrounding alveolar bone is illustrated. Highlighted here are the principal fibers of the periodontal ligament, which extend from the cementum to the alveolar bone. Note the interradicular fibers, which radiate from the crest of the interradicular bone to the cementum that lines the root furcation.

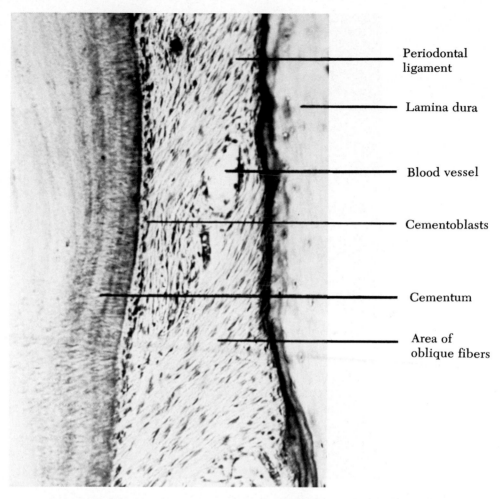

Periodontal ligament

Lamina dura

Blood vessel

Cementoblasts

Cementum

Area of oblique fibers

Figure 8–13. Photomicrograph of a human periodontal ligament and adjacent tissues, cut through the region of the oblique principal fiber bundles. Note the more coronal attachment of these fiber bundles to the bone. Coronal part of the tooth is at the top.

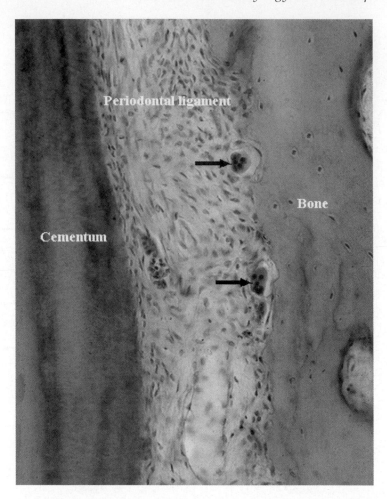

Figure 8–14. (See Color Plate) Photomicrograph of the periodontal ligament between cementum and lamina dura (bone). The arrows indicate two large multinucleate osteoclasts that are in resorption sites along the surface of the lamina dura. Can you identify other cell types? See Figs. 8-5 and 8-13.

fibers are usually not named in the arbitrary classification that has been given to the periodontal ligament fibers, they function with the previously described horizontal fibers to stabilize the tooth.

Apical fibers radiate around the apex of the tooth. At approximately right angles to their attachment in the cementum, they extend to their attachment in the bone at the bottom of the alveolus. Figures 8-1, 8-6, and 8-11 demonstrate that these apical fibers resist any force that tends to lift the tooth from the socket and function with the fibers of other groups to stabilize the tooth against forces that tend to produce a tilting movement.

Interradicular fibers are in the root furcation. They radiate from the crest of the interradicular septum to the cementum that lines the root furcation (Figs. 8-6 and 8-14). Interradicular fibers function to stabilize the tooth.

Scattered among the principal fibers of the periodontal ligament are smaller fibers that have no distinct orientation.

OTHER COMPONENTS OF THE PERIODONTAL LIGAMENT

Blood vessels of the periodontal ligament are branches of the superior or inferior alveolar artery and vein. They enter the periodontal ligament at various locations: at the fundus (bottom) of the alveolus, along with vessels that supply the tooth pulp; through openings in the bone of the sides of the alveolus, coming from the bone marrow spaces; and from the deeper branches of gingival blood vessels that pass over the alveolar crest.

Lymphatic vessels follow the path of the blood vessels.

Nerves of the periodontal ligament also generally follow the blood vessels. They are sensory nerves from the second division (in the maxilla) or the third division (in the mandible) of the fifth cranial nerve. They provide a sense of touch; that is, they enable the individual to be aware of a touch or tap given to the tooth.

Rests of Malassez, also called epithelial rests, are small groups of epithelial cells that are seen in microscopic examination of the periodontal ligament (Figs. 8-15 and 8-16). When such epithelial cells are seen microscopically as strings of cells rather than as round groups of cells in the periodontal ligament, they are referred to as remains of *Hertwig's epithelial root sheath* (see Figs. 3-31 and 3-32). Regardless

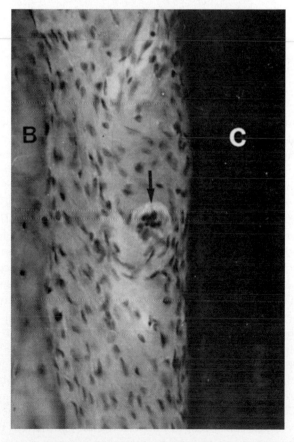

Figure 8–15. Microscopic view of an epithelial rest of Malassez (arrow) in the periodontal ligament, close to the cementum (C) and at a distance from the bone (B) of the socket. Most of the other cells scattered through the periodontal ligament are fibroblasts.

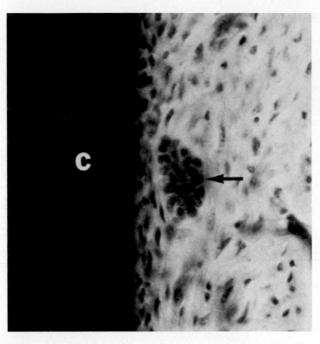

Figure 8–16. Higher magnification of an epithelial rest (arrow). Individual epithelial cells are clearly seen. Notice the most common position of the epithelial rest next to the cementum (C). Cemento-blasts are seen along the periodontal ligament surface of the cementum. Most of the other cells in the periodontal ligament are fibroblasts.

of the named used to refer to them, these epithelial cells found in the periodontal ligament have come to be recognized as cells derived from the enamel organ, which produced the tooth enamel during tooth formation (see Chapter 3). Their presence may be important pathologically in the formation of certain tumors and cyst linings.

Cementicles are minute calcified bodies sometimes seen in microscopic examination of the periodontal ligament of older individuals (Figs. 8-17 and 8-18). Cementicles may be attached to the cementum or may be entirely separate from the tooth root. Although their size varies, their shape is ordinarily spherical. Usually, cementicles are not considered to be of clinical importance.

Osteoblasts (osteo = bone; blasts = germ) are specialized connective tissue cells found at the surface of bone, where bone formation is occurring. They may be seen in the periodontal ligament at the surface of the bone of the tooth socket, where bone is being laid down (Fig. 8-5). Osteoclasts (clast = break) are specialized connective tissue cells that border bone that is being resorbed. They may occur in the periodontal ligament next to the bone of the tooth socket, where bone resorption is taking place (Figs. 8-14 and 8-19). Similarly, cementoblasts (Figs. 8-5 and 8-13) are specialized connective tissue cells that accompany cementum formation, and cementoclasts are specialized connective tissue cells that accompany cementum resorption. These cells occur in the periodontal ligament at the surface of the cementum, where cementum formation or cementum resorption is taking place. (See Chapter 9.)

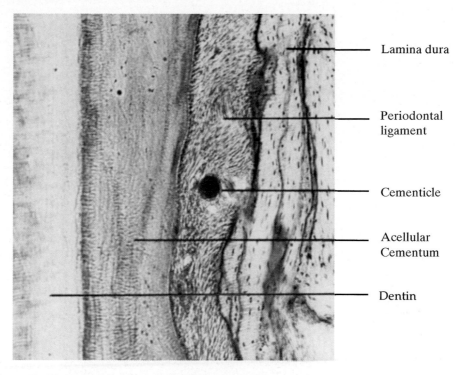

Lamina dura

Periodontal
ligament

Cementicle

Acellular
Cementum

Dentin

Figure 8–17. Photomicrograph of a section through a human tooth and its adjacent tissues. A cementicle is seen surrounded by periodontal ligament tissue.

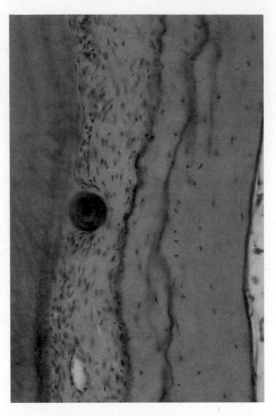

Figure 8–18. (See Color Plates) Microscopic view of normal-appearing cementum, periodontal ligament, and alveolar bone. Of interest is the cementicle attached to the cementum.

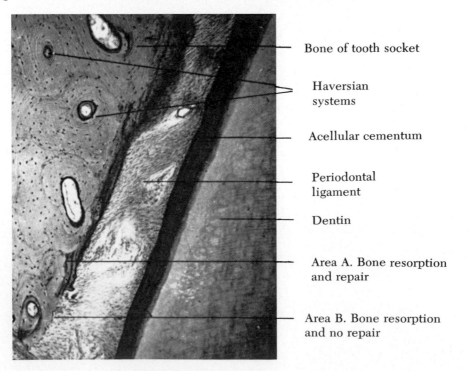

Bone of tooth socket

Haversian systems

Acellular cementum

Periodontal ligament

Dentin

Area A. Bone resorption and repair

Area B. Bone resorption and no repair

FUNCTIONS AND CLINICAL IMPORTANCE OF THE PERIODONTAL LIGAMENT

The functions of the periodontal ligament may be described as supportive, formative, resorptive, sensory, and nutritive.

The *supportive function* of the periodontal ligament results from the ingenious arrangement of its principal fibers. These fibers are so arranged that functional pressure on the tooth crown from any direction produces a tension of certain fiber groups. Consequently, pressure on the tooth crown is transmitted to the bone of the tooth socket and to the cementum as a pull. Because of this fiber arrangement that suspends the tooth in its socket, the tooth is not pressed against the bone of the socket wall during the process of biting and chewing. However, a sudden, excessive pressure applied to a tooth crown, such as an accidental blow, may damage the periodontal ligament sufficiently to loosen the tooth.

The sturdy principal fibers of the periodontal ligament that separate the cementum of the tooth root from the wall of the socket by less than 0.25 mm are able to withstand the heavy force produced by the powerful jaw muscles. A study of 53 young adults at the School of Dentistry in Melbourne, Australia, showed the average biting force for men to be 19.6 kgf (kilograms force) for anterior teeth and 29.3 kgf for posterior teeth (43 pounds and 65 pounds, respectively); for women, the average biting force was 13.5 kgf for anterior teeth and 21.3 kgf for posterior teeth (30 pounds and 47 pounds, respectively).

The *formative function* of the periodontal ligament is seen in both developing teeth and in adult functioning teeth. During tooth development, cells of the periodontal ligament produce both the cementum of the tooth root and the bone of the tooth socket. In the functioning tooth, cementoblasts of the periodontal ligament are able to produce cementum at any time during the life of the tooth; its osteoblasts maintain the bone of the tooth socket by producing new bone following bone resorption (Figs. 8-13, 8-14, and 8-19). The fibroblasts of the periodontal ligament produce the collagen and ground substance, which are subject to a dynamic turnover, especially during orthodontic treatment. Evidence shows that fibroblasts may also play a role in the lysis or dissolution of collagen fibers. When they perform this function, they are referred to as *fibroclasts*.

The *resorptive function* of the periodontal ligament accompanies the formative function. Whereas tension (pull) on the periodontal ligament fibers tends to stimulate cementum and bone formation, pressure stimulates bone resorption. Severe pressure produces rapid bone resorption and sometimes may also result in resorption of the more resistant cementum. If the pressure is sufficiently severe, it may destroy areas of the periodontal ligament. The processes of bone formation and resorption are treated more thoroughly in the review of bone and the alveolar process (see Chapter 9).

The *sensory function* of the periodontal ligament is seen in the ability of an individual to estimate the amount of pressure in mastication and to identify which of several teeth receives a slight tap with an instrument.

The *nutritive function* is served by the presence of blood vessels in the periodontal ligament.

Figure 8–19. Photomicrograph of a small area of tooth root with the associated periodontal ligament and lamina dura. The direction of the periodontal ligament fibers shows that the crown of the tooth was at the bottom of the pictured area. Notice the resorption of the alveolar bone (B). Bone resorption (A) reached as far as the end of the pointer line, and then bone apposition (addition) occurred on the surface of the resorbed area (repair).

Without the periodontal ligament, a tooth could not be retained in its socket. Localized destruction of the periodontal ligament may be repaired by the formation of new tissue after the cause of the destruction has been removed. Localized detachment from the cementum of the principal fibers of the periodontal ligament may be followed by fiber reattachment if removal of irritating factors permits the formation of new cementum. Extensive destruction of the periodontal ligament may necessitate removal of the tooth.

SUGGESTED READING

Atkinson HF, Ralph WJ. Tooth loss and biting force in man. J Dent Res 1973;52:225–228.

Schroeder HE, Listgarten MA. The gingival tissues: the architecture of periodontal protection. Periodontol 2000 1997;13:91–120.

Ten Cate AR, Mills C, Solomon G. The development of the periodontium. A transplantation and autoradiograph study. Anat Rec 1971;170:365–379.

Bone and the Alveolar Processes

BONE

The word *bone* is used to designate both an organ and a tissue. As a tissue, a bone is one of the connective tissues and is composed of osteocytes (bone cells) and an organic matrix that mineralizes. A bone that is an organ, such as the mandible, is composed of bone tissue. Bone tissue contains bone marrow in its center and has a close association with blood vessels and nerves.

GROSS STRUCTURE OF A BONE (ORGAN)

Although bones appear to be solid organs, they are not completely solid structures. The bone tissue of which bones are composed may be described as *compact bone* and *trabecular bone* (or *spongy bone*). The outside wall of a bone is compact bone. Each bone also has a hollow center, the *bone marrow cavity*, into which *trabeculae* (bars or plates) of bone protrude. These trabeculae make up trabecular bone. In the spaces around the trabeculae in the bone marrow cavity is the *bone marrow*.

Examine Figures 9-1 (a drawing of a faciolingual section of a human mandible), 9-2 (a faciolingual section through a mandibular premolar), 9-3 (a faciolingual histologic section of an edentulous human mandible), and 9-4 (a drawing of a mesiodistal section of a mandible). Notice the compact character of the bone that makes up the outer wall of the mandible and the trabeculae that project into the marrow cavity. The number and size of the trabeculae in the marrow cavity of a bone are determined to a large degree by the functional activity of the organ: the greater the functional activity, the greater the number of trabeculae.

Certain advantages result from this arrangement of bone tissue into compact and trabecular bone. First, a large bone with trabeculae and bone marrow in its center weighs much less than would a similar organ composed of solid bone tissue. Second, bone marrow makes the nutrition provided by the blood vessels located both inside the organ and on its outside surface available to the bone tissue.

The outside surface of all bones is covered by a thin connective tissue membrane called the *periosteum* (peri = around; osteum = bone). The inside surfaces of bones are covered with a much more delicate connective tissue membrane called the *endosteum* (endo = within) (Fig. 9-1).

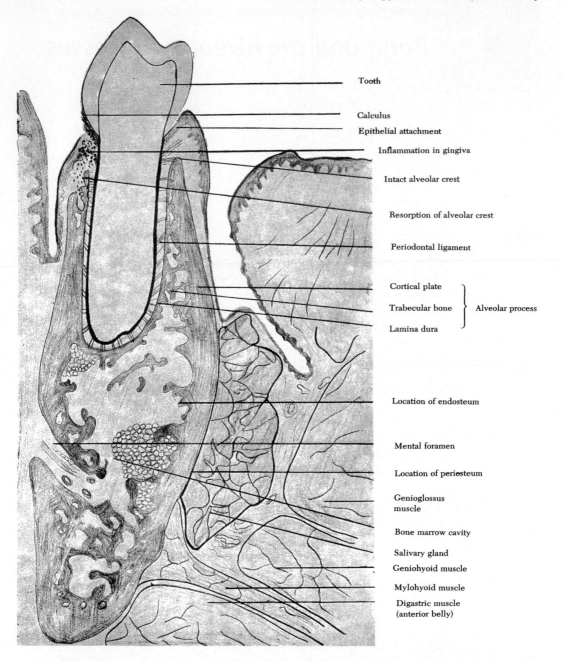

Tooth

Calculus

Epithelial attachment

Inflammation in gingiva

Intact alveolar crest

Resorption of alveolar crest

Periodontal ligament

Cortical plate

Trabecular bone   } Alveolar process

Lamina dura

Location of endosteum

Mental foramen

Location of periosteum

Genioglossus
muscle

Bone marrow cavity

Salivary gland

Geniohyoid muscle

Mylohyoid muscle

Digastric muscle
(anterior belly)

Figure 9–1. Diagrammatic drawing of a faciolingual section of a human mandible in the region of the second premolar (much enlarged). This section is not cut through the pulp cavity of the tooth.

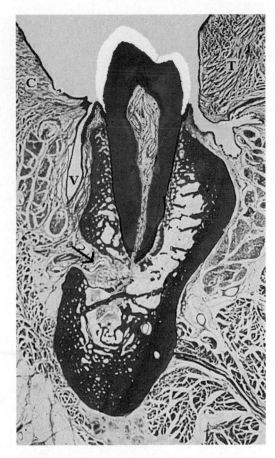

Figure 9–2. (See Color Plates) Faciolingual section of a human mandible in the region of the second premolar. C, cheek; T, tongue; V, facial vestibule. The arrow is in the mental foramen. How many areas can you identify by referring to Fig. 9-1?

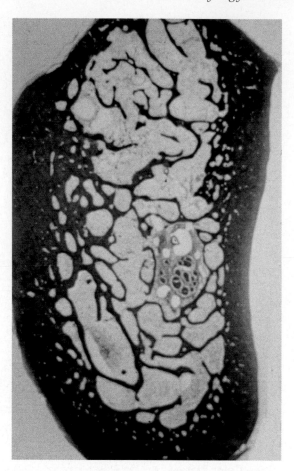

Figure 9–3. Faciolingual histologic section of an edentulous human mandible. The compact bone tissue on the outside is continuous with trabecular (spongy) bone tissue on the inside. The open spaces between the trabecular bone are the sites of the bone marrow tissue. A cross section of the inferior alveolar canal is surrounded by trabecular bone (mid-right). Notice the outline of the inferior alveolar nerve and blood vessels in the canal.

Figure 9–4. Diagrammatic drawing of a section of a human mandible bearing an isolated first molar tooth, cut mesiodistally. 1. Pulp horn. 2. Gingival fibers of periodontal ligament. 3. Bone of interradicular septum (between the roots). 4. Cortical bone on ridge of mandible. 5. Lamina dura bone near apex of distal root. 6. Cross section of small blood vessel. 7. Fat marrow. 8. Trabecular bone scattered throughout bone marrow cavity. 9. Longitudinal section of blood vessel. 10. Inferior alveolar nerve. 11. Cortical bone on inferior surface of mandible.

A, B, C, and D indicate different areas of the periodontal ligament. A. The periodontal ligament on the mesial side of the mesial root. B. The periodontal ligament on the mesial side of the distal root. At both A and B, the principal fibers have a wavy appearance, and evidence of resorption of the lamina dura bone is evident. C. The periodontal ligament on the distal side of the mesial root. D. The periodontal ligament on the distal side of the distal root. At C and D, the principal fibers are straight, and resorption of the lamina dura is not evident. Perhaps this tooth was undergoing a slight movement in a mesial direction; the slight pressure on the mesial side of each root resulted in relaxed periodontal ligament fibers and in bone resorption in the lamina dura. On the distal side of each root, the fibers are straight, and bone resorption is not evident. The interradicular fibers of the periodontal ligament radiate from the crest of the interradicular septum to the cementum that lines the root furcation.

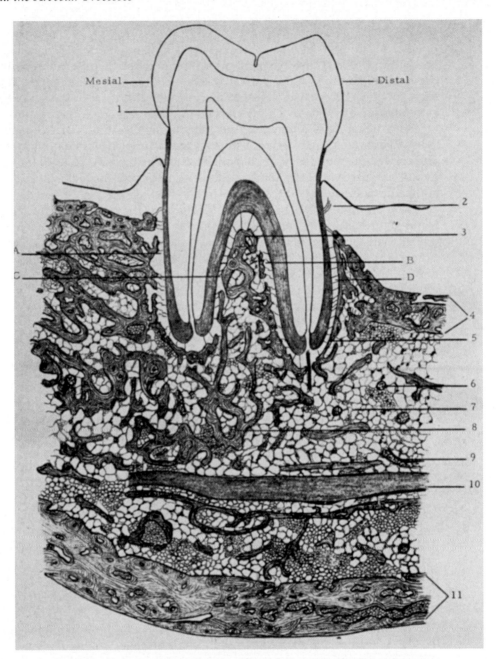

MICROSCOPIC STRUCTURE OF BONE (TISSUE)

Bone tissue consists of bone cells and a bone matrix, which is made of fibrous and ground types of intercellular substance. Because the intercellular substance becomes mineralized, bone is a hard tissue. Bone is approximately 50% mineral substance and 50% organic substance and water. It has about the same hardness as cementum.

As is true for dentin and cementum, chemically the fibrous type of intercellular substance is collagen; the ground substance is a complex of mucopolysaccharides. The crystalline (inorganic) part of bone is similar to that of enamel, dentin, and cementum-hydroxyapatite crystals. Table 9-1, compares bone to the other three mineralized tissues of the body.

Osteocytes (osteo = bone; cyte = cell), which are the cells of bone tissue, are distributed throughout the mineralized intercellular substance. The space in the bone matrix that is occupied by an osteocyte is called a *lacuna* (little space) (Figs. 9-5, 9-6, and 9-7). Lacunae are connected to one another by a system of *canaliculi* (little canals). These canaliculi extend not only from one lacuna to another, but some of them also open into the various canals of bone in which capillaries are located. Tissue fluids pass from the capillaries to the canaliculi and, therefore, from one lacuna to another throughout the bone tissue (Figs. 9-8 and 9-9).

Mature bone tissue is formed in thin layers called *lamellae*. Lamellae have two distinct patterns of arrangement, and, according to their pattern, bone tissue is called either *Haversian system bone* or *lamellar bone*.

In Haversian system bone, the lamellae are arranged in concentric circles around a small central canal, which is called an *Haversian canal*. The canal contains capillary-like blood vessels that are surrounded by a loose, soft tissue, which is referred to as *perivascular connective tissue*. A series of concentric lamellae with the included Haversian canal is called an *Haversian system* (Figs. 9-5, 9-6, 9-7, and 9-8). An Haversian system may contain from 4 to 20 concentric lamellae and measures approximately 0.1 mm in diameter.

In *lamellar bone*, which makes up the outside surface of most bones, the lamellae are not arranged in small concentric circles, but follow the surface, or circumference, of the bone. In this location, the lamellar bone is sometimes given the additional names of *circumferential bone* or *subperiosteal bone* (sub = below; periosteal = of the periosteum). Lamellar bone also often makes up the surfaces of the trabeculae of trabecular bone; in this location, it may be called *subendosteal bone*. Both the Haversian system bone and lamellar bone are found in all mature human bones (Figs. 9-5, 9-8, and 9-9).

Regardless of the arrangement of bone lamellae, bone tissue contains osteocytes that lie in lacunae and connect through canaliculi. This system of connected bone cells (Figs. 9-6 and 9-9) is the means by which nutrients are distributed throughout the bone tissue. In an Haversian system, some of the canaliculi open into the Haversian canal, thereby providing a pathway by which nutrients from the blood vessels contained in the canal may reach the osteocytes of the Haversian system.

Bone is a vascular tissue and, therefore, contains many blood vessels. Arteries and veins enter and leave a bone in various places, both from the outside surface and from the bone marrow cavity. The canals in a bone through which blood vessels pass into the bone tissue from the outside of the organ or from the bone mar-

TABLE 9–1. Comparison of the Four Mineralized Tissues

	Enamel	Dentin	Cementum	Bone
Embryonic tissue origin	Lining epithelium[a]	Mesenchyme	Mesenchyme	Mesenchyme
Matrix-forming cell	Ameloblast	Odontoblast	Cementoblast	Osteoblast
Growth mechanism	Appositional	Appositional	Appositional	Appositional
Organic material Fibrous	Amelogenins, enamelins[a]	Collagen	Collagen	Collagen
Ground substance	Mucopolysaccharide	Mucopolysaccharide	Mucopolysaccharide	Mucopolysaccharide
Tissue Fluid	Present	Present	Present	Present
Internal cellular elements	None[a]	Cell processes	Cellular: Cells, processes Acellular: none	Cells, processes
Internal cellular space	None[a]	Tubules	Cellular: lacunae, canaliculi Acellular: none	Lacunae and canaliculi
Internal vascular space	None	None	None	Present[a]
Adjacent "free" surface environment	Saliva[a]	Pulp[b]	Periodontal ligament[b]	Periosteum, endosteum[b]

[a] Denotes differences.
[b] Connective tissue.

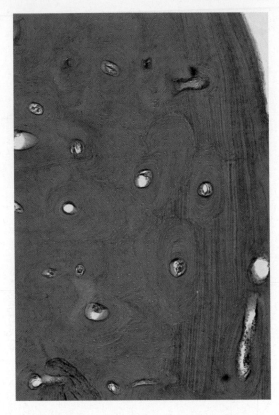

Figure 9–5. (See Color Plates) Photomicrograph of a demineralized section of compact bone tissue of a human mandible. Cross sections of Haversian systems are present, as are the lacunae that contain cell bodies of osteocytes; circumferential lamellae of the outer surface are also seen (right). See Fig. 9-9 for a diagrammatic interpretation of the vascular canals of compact bone.

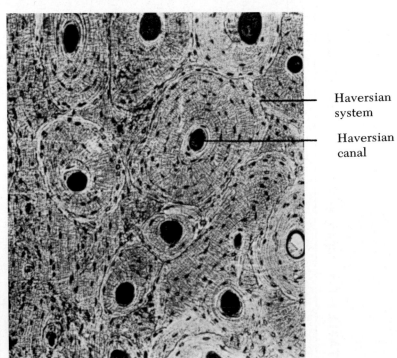

Haversian
system

Haversian
canal

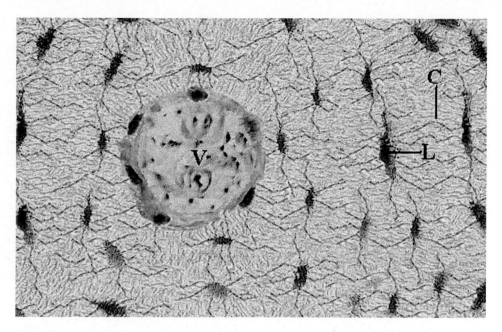

Figure 9–7. Photomicrograph of an Haversian system, cut in cross section on a ground histologic section (high power). The diameter of an Haversian system is approximately 0.1 mm. Note the relation of the lacuna (L), which is site of the osteocyte cell body, to the canaliculi (C), which are the sites of the osteocyte cell processes, and to the vascular canal (V), which is the site of blood vessels, nerves, and osteogenic connective tissue.

Figure 9–6. Photomicrograph of a ground cross section of a dried, undecalcified piece of bone from a human clavicle. Cross sections of several Haversian systems are present. The concentric lamellae and lacunae of the Haversian systems are clear. In the center of each Haversian system is the Haversian canal. Notice the size of the many small lacunae compared to that of the larger Haversian vascular canals. On close inspection, tiny canaliculi can be seen radiating from the lacunae. See Fig. 9-7 for a higher magnification of an Haversian system.

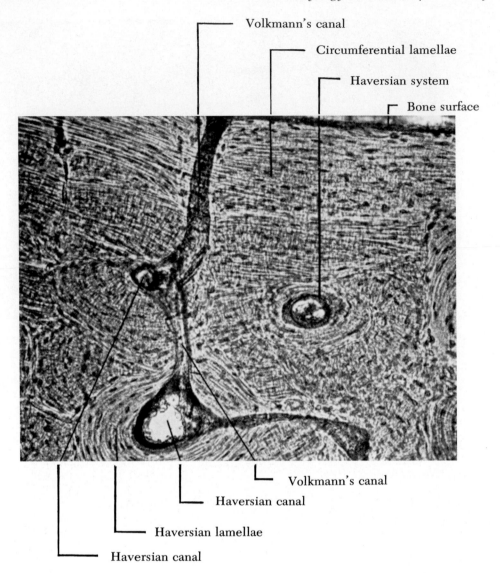

Volkmann's canal

Circumferential lamellae

Haversian system

Bone surface

Volkmann's canal

Haversian canal

Haversian lamellae

Haversian canal

Figure 9–8. Photomicrograph of a ground section of a human femur. The surface of the bone is seen (upper right). A Volkmann's canal cuts through the surface circumferential lamellae and enters an Haversian canal slightly (left of center). The Volkmann's canal continues (bottom) to a second Haversian canal (note the concentric bone lamellae around the canal). The Volkmann's canal then turns right (across bottom of picture). By such a route, blood vessels and nerves supply bone tissue.

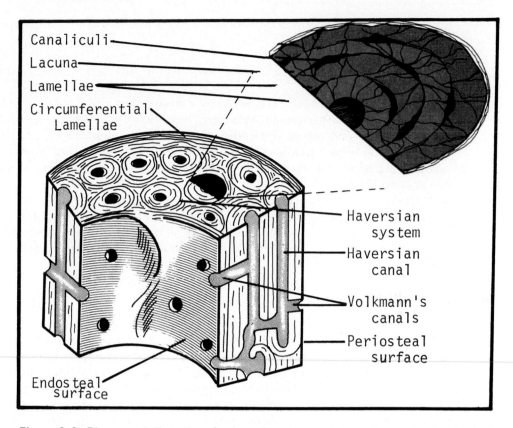

Figure 9–9. Diagrammatic illustration of a piece of long bone, cut to reveal a cross section, longitudinal section of the organ, and the wall of the bone marrow cavity. The holes in the marrow cavity wall are openings of canals that carry blood vessels between the bone marrow and bone tissue. On the longitudinal surface of the bone, canals lie longitudinally in the organ and have horizontal branches from one long canal to another and from long canals to the marrow cavity. The crosscut surface reveals cross sections of the long canals, each surrounded by several bone lamellae. Each Haversian canal and its several lamellae constitute an Haversian system. On this surface are also the circumferential lamellae that constitute the outer surface of the organ.

An enlargement of half of a cross section of a single Haversian system shows the Haversian canal surrounded by several Haversian lamellae. Between the lamellae are lacunae that housed osteocytes in the living bone. The lacunae are connected to one another and the Haversian canal by numerous canaliculi.

row cavity are called *Volkmann's canals* (Figs. 9-8 and 9-9). Branches of the blood vessels contained in Volkmann's canals enter the smaller Haversian canals.

It seems remarkable that blood vessels should enter and be distributed throughout bones as they are; however, during the embryonic development of the body, the larger blood vessels are formed and in place before bone formation begins. As bone is formed, it simply surrounds and encloses any blood vessels located in the area. Therefore, blood vessels can enter and leave bones at various points.

Bone marrow, which occupies the centers of bones in the spaces around the trabeculae, is a soft tissue (Figs. 9-1, 9-2, and 9-3). The two types of bone marrow are *red marrow*, which is found in most of the bones of young individuals and produces red and white blood cells, and *yellow marrow* (fat marrow), which does not have a blood-forming function. In adults, most red marrow becomes converted into yellow marrow. Only certain locations in the adult skeleton retain the red type of marrow that continues to perform the function of hemopoiesis (hemo = blood; poiesis = creation).

PERIOSTEUM AND ENDOSTEUM

The outside surface of a bone is covered by a more or less tough connective tissue membrane called the periosteum. A thinner, more delicate connective tissue membrane, called the endosteum, covers the inner surface of compact bone and the trabeculae in the bone marrow cavity and lines the Haversian and Volkmann's canals. The periosteum and endosteum function in both the formation and resorption of bone tissue.

The periodontal ligament, which surrounds the root of a tooth and separates it from the bone of the tooth socket, is a specialized periosteum. It functions on one side in the formation and resorption of the bone comprising the tooth socket and on the other side in the formation and resorption of the cementum covering the tooth root.

GROWTH OF BONE

Bone growth includes both *bone formation* and *bone resorption*.

Bone formation involves both the conversion of relatively unspecialized connective tissue into bone matrix and bone cells and the subsequent mineralization of the bone matrix. Bone matrix is composed of two kinds of intercellular substance: fibrous and ground substance. It arises as a result of a chemical change that takes place in the intercellular substances of unspecialized connective tissue. The bone cells also are cells of this connective tissue that become entrapped in the forming bone matrix.

In a growing bone, the connective tissue that forms the new bone is either the periosteum or endosteum, depending on whether the new bone is being added to the outside or the inside of the organ. The intercellular substance of the part of the periosteum (or endosteum) that lies against the bone surface is chemically changed into the bone matrix. Some of the cells of the periosteum (or endosteum) that are next to the bone surface become specialized and are called *osteoblasts* (osteo = bone; blast = germ) (Figs. 9-10, 9-11, 9-12, 9-13, and 9-14). Some osteoblasts become surrounded by the forming bone matrix and, therefore, become cells of the bone tissue called osteocytes (Figs. 9-6 and 9-14). Because the osteoblasts in the periosteum (or endosteum) are not completely isolated cells, but have their cytoplasm connected with other osteoblasts by numerous thin projections, the osteocytes likewise are not isolated cells, but have their cytoplasm connected with other osteocytes by the same thin projections (Fig. 9-9). The spaces in the bone matrix occupied by the osteocytes are the lacunae, and the spaces occupied by the numerous cytoplasmic connections are the canaliculi.

In the embryonic development of certain bones, the formation of bone tissue is preceded by the formation of a cartilage model that resembles the shape of the bone that is to be formed. This cartilage predecessor of the bone mineralizes and then is gradually removed by resorption. As the mineralized cartilage is resorbed, bone tissue is formed to replace it. Bones that arise in this way, with a cartilage structure preceding the development of bone tissue, are said to be formed by *en-*

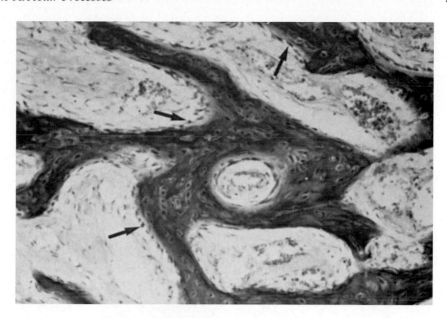

Figure 9–10. Microscopic view of a section of embryonic bone tissue of a mandible. Osteoblasts (arrows) are within the highly vascular mesenchymal tissue along the surfaces of the bone. This figure represents intramembranous bone formation.

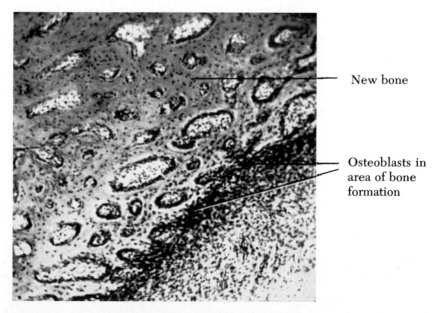

New bone

Osteoblasts in area of bone formation

Figure 9–11. Photomicrograph of a section of forming bone in the area of the mandible in a kitten fetus (medium power). Intramembranous bone formation is displayed. Osteoblasts are numerous, and the connective tissue from which the bone is forming can be seen (lower right).

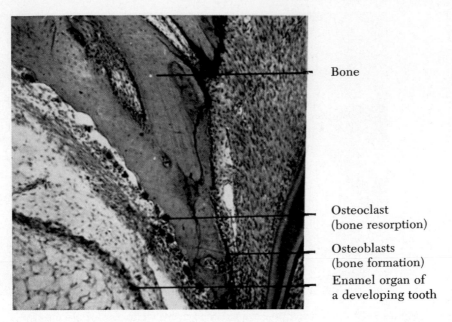

Bone

Osteoclast
(bone resorption)

Osteoblasts
(bone formation)

Enamel organ of
a developing tooth

Figure 9–12. Photomicrograph of a small area of kitten mandible in the region of developing teeth (low power). The large triangular piece of bone shows bone resorption on one side (left) and bone formation on the other (right). In the area of bone resorption are many osteoclasts on the bone surface. Resorption in this area is most likely the result of the presence of a developing tooth, the enamel organ of which is seen (lower left). On the right side of the triangular bone, the presence of numerous, closely packed osteoblasts on the bone surface is associated with formation of bone tissue in this area.

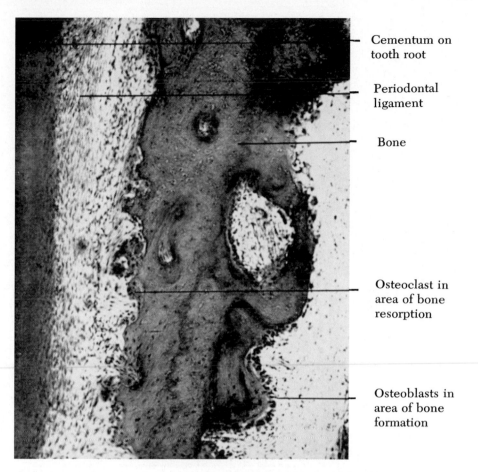

Cementum on
tooth root

Periodontal
ligament

Bone

Osteoclast in
area of bone
resorption

Osteoblasts in
area of bone
formation

Figure 9–13. Photomicrograph of an area of tooth root, periodontal ligament, and alveolar bone or lamina dura (medium power). This tooth was not functional. Notice the lack of orientation of periodontal ligament fibers. Bone resorption occurs on the bone surface, next to the periodontal ligament. Notice the osteoclasts. On the outer surface of the bone (right), the presence of osteoblasts indicates bone formation.

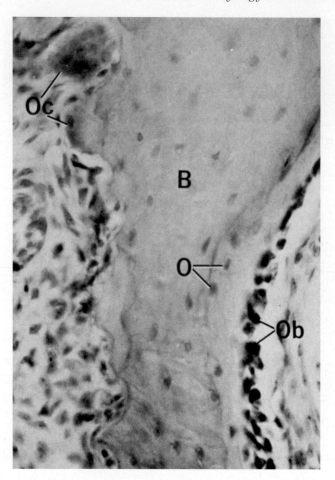

Figure 9–14. Higher magnification of an area of bone (B) shows resorption (left) by osteoclasts (OC) and formation (right) by osteoblasts (OB). O, osteocytes.

dochondral formation (Fig. 9-15). Examples of bones formed in this manner are the long bones of the arms and legs.

In the embryonic development of other bones, the bone tissue is formed without a preceding cartilage pattern, and these bones are said to be formed by *intramembranous formation* (Figs. 9-10 and 9-11). Examples of bones formed in this manner, with no preceding cartilage structure, are the mandible and maxillae. The process of the conversion of unspecialized connective tissue into bone and the final microscopic structure of bone tissue are the same whether or not bone formation has been preceded by cartilage.

Although at first glance bone appears to be a permanent and unchanging tissue, it is in a state of constant change. Bone tissue formation continues practically throughout the life of the bone, but the organ does not become indefinitely heavier and greater in mass. The density and size of a bone are limited because the formation of bone tissue in one place is compensated for by the resorption of bone tissue in another.

Bone resorption is the removal of both the mineral materials and organic matrix of bone. Resorption of bone should not be confused with demineralization of bone (or other hard tissues), such as occurs when the tissue is removed from the body and taken to the laboratory to be placed in a weak acid solution. In this laboratory procedure, called demineralization, the mineral material is removed, and the organic material remains. In bone resorption, the organic matrix and the mineral material are both removed, and nothing of the bone remains.

Bone resorption occurs just beneath the periosteum or endosteum. A specialized type of cell called an *osteoclast* (clast = break) is associated with the resorption of bone tissue (Figs. 9-12 and 9-13). Osteoclasts are multinucleated cells that contain from 1 to 3 dozen nuclei in a single cell (Fig. 9-16).

The processes of bone formation and resorption occur in all bones intermittently throughout the life of an individual. The intramembranous bone (Fig. 9-10) and endochondral bone (Fig. 9-15) that form in the early development of the individual are gradually resorbed and replaced by mature bone. With growth and function, mature bone undergoes an endless process of resorption in one place and apposition (formation) in another (Fig. 9-14). Haversian systems are partially or wholly resorbed and then replaced by other Haversian systems or by lamellar bone. Lamellar bone is resorbed and replaced by Haversian system bone or by new lamellar bone. This turnover is rapid during the growth of the individual and oc-

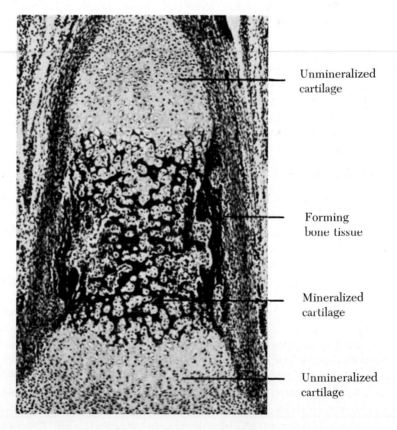

Unmineralized cartilage

Forming bone tissue

Mineralized cartilage

Unmineralized cartilage

Figure 9–15. Photomicrograph of a section of a developing bone from the foot of a human fetus. Endochondral bone formation is displayed. The ends of the organ are cartilage that is not yet calcified. The center portion has areas of mineralized cartilage which appear dark in the picture. The unmineralized cartilage gradually calcifies and is resorbed and replaced by bone tissue. Forming bone tissue is present at the outer surface of the mineralized cartilage.

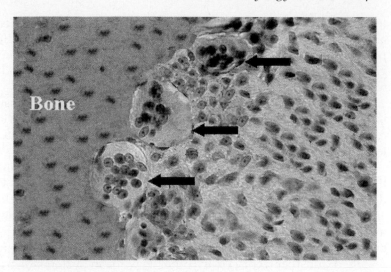

Figure 9–16. Arrows point to large, multinucleated osteoclasts.

curs more slowly later in life. After full individual growth has been attained, however, the processes of bone change may continue to occur rapidly in places where function or trauma stimulate resorption or apposition.

Bone formation and resorption take place continuously in response to certain stimuli in some areas of the bone tissue that surrounds the teeth. In the tooth socket, the stimuli that govern bone formation and bone resorption are tension (pull) on the periodontal ligament fibers attached to the bone and pressure on the periodontal ligament and bone. Tension on the periodontal ligament fibers induces bone formation; pressure induces bone resorption.

THE ALVEOLAR PROCESS

The *alveolar process* is defined as the part of the mandible and maxillae that surrounds and supports the teeth (Figs. 9-1, 9-17, and 9-18). The alveolar process supports the tooth roots on the facial, palatal, and lingual sides; extends between the teeth, separating them on the mesial and distal sides; and extends into the furcation of the roots of multirooted teeth (Figs. 9-1, 9-4, and 9-19). The occlusal border of the alveolar process, which is located near the cervix of the tooth, is referred to as the *alveolar crest*.

The alveolar process may be described as being composed of the lamina dura[1] and supporting bone. The lamina dura is the bone of the wall of the tooth socket. The supporting bone is made of the cortical plate, which is the outside wall of the mandible and maxillae, and the trabecular bone, which in many areas is located between the lamina dura and the cortical bone (Figs. 9-4 and 9-20). In some areas, the alveolar process is thin and contains little or no trabecular bone, and the lamina dura and cortical plate are fused. This kind of thin alveolar process is found, among other places, on the facial surfaces of mandibular anterior teeth.

---

[1] Also called *alveolar bone, true alveolar bone, alveolar bone proper*, and *cribriform plate*.

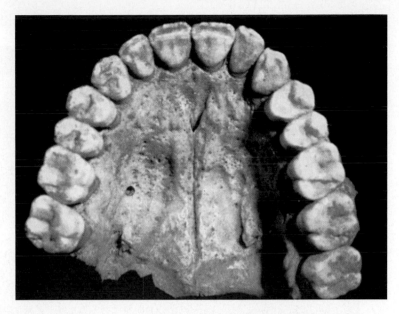

Figure 9–17. A human maxilla. The palatal part of the alveolar process merges without a distinct line into the bone of the palate. The alveolar process extending between the teeth is seen clearly. The alveolar crest is the edge of the alveolar process around the cervix of the tooth. Notice the attrition of the incisal edges of the anterior teeth.

Maxillary third molar

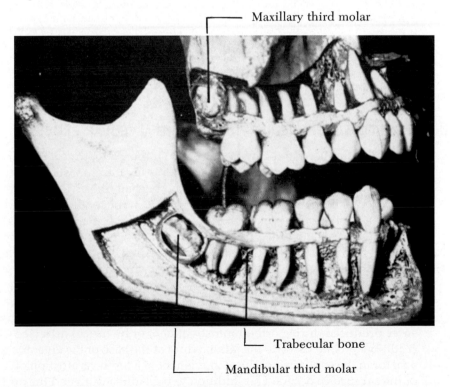

Trabecular bone

Mandibular third molar

Figure 9–18. A human maxilla and mandible with the facial parts of the alveolar process removed, except in the area of the cervical border. In the mandible, some trabecular bone remains among the tooth roots. Notice the location and position of the developing mandibular and maxillary third molars. The crown of the mandibular third molar is nearly completed in the ramus of the mandible. Its occlusal surface is directed mesially and occlusally, and it is surrounded by a bony crypt. The maxillary third molar is directed buccally and distally.

213

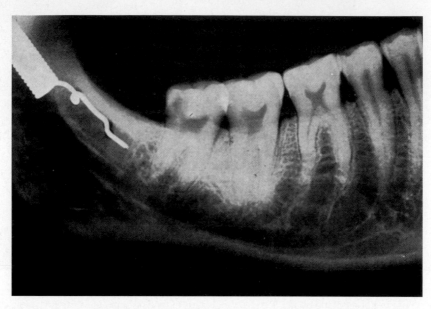

Figure 9–19. Radiograph of a human mandible similar to that in Fig. 9-17. The third molar is erupted, and the roots appear to be fully formed. The trabeculae in the interradicular bone (between the roots) and the interdental bone (between the teeth) have a characteristic orientation, and many are positioned horizontally. The space occupied by the periodontal ligament is seen here most clearly on the distal side of the distal root of the first molar. In the ramus of the mandible, and extending beneath the tooth roots, is the mandibular canal. The locations at which branches from the mandibular nerve extended from the mandibular canal to the apical foramina of the first molar roots are visible in the bone pattern. The white object (left) is a spring that attached the mandible to the temporal bone of the prepared skull. (Courtesy Dr. Richard C. O'Brien, College of Dentistry, Ohio State University.)

CLINICAL ASPECTS OF BONE REACTION IN THE ALVEOLAR PROCESS

The trabecular bone and lamina dura that support a tooth react in different ways to changes in tooth function. When a tooth is in strong masticatory function, the trabecular bone in the alveolar process and beneath the alveolus[2] of the tooth are composed of numerous heavy bone trabeculae. If the tooth is removed from function by loss of opposing teeth, these supporting trabeculae become less numerous and smaller. When the tooth in question is again placed in occlusion by the replacement of the lost teeth in the opposing arch, trabecular bone again forms around the tooth that has resumed masticatory function.

The lamina dura (Fig. 9-21) does not respond by resorption to loss of masticatory function of the tooth. However, it may respond by resorption to various stimuli, such as trauma that results from faulty occlusion, periodontal disease, pressures produced during orthodontic treatment or by mesial drift (see Chapter 12). Addition of bone tissue to the lamina dura at the base of the alveolus also may be a factor in the continued occlusal movement of a tooth, as attrition on the occlusal or incisal surface occurs. This addition to the lamina dura and the addition of cementum to the root may partially compensate for loss of crown length caused by attrition.

---

[2]Pronounced *ăl vē' ō lŭs* (the tooth socket).

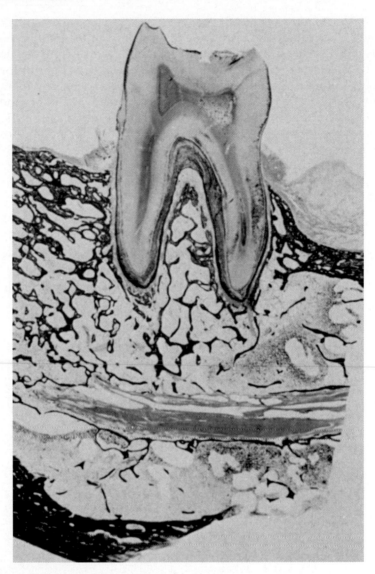

Figure 9–20. Histologic section through a mandibular first molar and its alveolar process. For a detailed description, see diagram of this section in Fig. 9-4. The enamel of the tooth was lost during histologic preparation.

Inflammation and swelling of the soft tissues around a tooth may result in damage to the periodontal ligament and resorption of the crest of the alveolar process (Figs. 9-1 and 11-13). The presence of calculus in the gingival sulcus has the potential to set off a series of events: the calculus serves as a nidus for microorganisms that produce inflammation and swelling of the adjacent soft tissues. This condition involves and damages the periodontal ligament fibers around the neck of the tooth. Damage to the periodontal ligament results in resorption of the bone to which the fibers are attached, and continued inflammation produces continued bone resorption. Eventually, so much damage may be done to the periodontal ligament and lamina dura that removal of the tooth becomes necessary.

Good oral hygiene and prompt dental care prevent such serious involvement because of the following consequential reactions.

1. Removal of the calculus may be expected to result in the elimination of the inflammation and swelling.
2. Elimination of the inflammation and swelling permits repair of the periodontal ligament.
3. Concurrently, resorption of the bone of the alveolar crest is arrested.
4. Additional cementum may be produced on the tooth root in the affected area

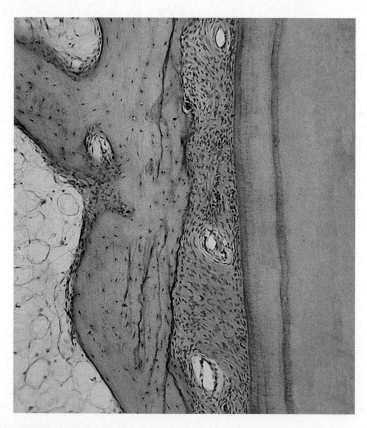

Figure 9–21. (See Color Plates) From left to right, a microscopic view of the lamina dura (compact bone) of the alveolar process, periodontal ligament, and tooth root. Note the many cells enclosed within both the bone and periodontal ligament in contrast to the obviously acellular cementum. Two sites of yellow bone marrow (fat cells) are present (far left).

with an accompanying reattachment of the previously damaged periodontal ligament.

5. Repair of some of the resorbed areas of the lamina dura may occur, and some bone construction may take place on the alveolar crest. The alveolar crest may occupy a position apical to that of the original position; that is, bone replacement on the alveolar crest will not be sufficient to restore the crest to its original height.

By accident or design, teeth are sometimes subject to pressure on the crown from a horizontal direction (Figs. 9-4 and 9-20). When the pressure is continued but not severe enough to damage the periodontal ligament, an adaptive response is produced in the lamina dura. On the side of the tooth socket toward which the tooth is pushed, the periodontal ligament and lamina dura are subject to pressures, and bone resorption occurs. On the side of the tooth socket away from which the tooth is pulled, the periodontal ligament fibers are subject to tension, and additional bone of the lamina dura is formed. The result of this bone resorption and bone formation is a change in the location of both the tooth socket and the tooth.

Such a change in the position of a tooth may result from change in occlusal pressures or may be a consequence of treatment applied by an orthodontist to improve unsatisfactory tooth alignment. The orthodontist places appliances on a patient's teeth and adjusts them at intervals to maintain proper pressures and tensions. Teeth that are being treated actually change location in the mouth. The success of this treatment is the result of three factors: bone is resorbed more easily than is cementum, the area of the lamina dura toward which the tooth is moved is resorbed, and the area of the lamina dura away from which the tooth is moved is built up.

SUGGESTED READINGS

Barbour SE, Nakashima K, Zhang JB, et al. Tobacco and smoking: environmental factors that modify the host response (immune system) and have an impact on periodontal health. Crit Rev Oral Biol Med 1997;8:437–460.

Jeffcoat MK. Osteoporosis: a possible modifying factor in oral bone loss. Ann Periodontol 1998;3:312–321.

Saffar JL, Lasfargues JJ, Cherruau M. Alveolar bone and the alveolar process: the socket that is never stable. Periodontol 2000 1997;13:76–90.

Schwartz Z, Goultschin J, Dean DD, Boyan BD. Mechanisms of alveolar bone destruction in periodontitis. Periodontol 2000 1997;14:158–172.

Zernik JH, Nowroozi N, Liu YH, Maxson R. Development, maturation, and aging of the alveolar bone. New insights. Dent Clin North Am 1997;41:1–15.

10   *The Oral Mucous Membranes*

MUCOUS MEMBRANES

Definition

A mucous membrane is the lining of a body cavity that opens to the outside of the body. Mucous membranes line the oral and nasal cavities, the sinuses, the trachea, the stomach and intestines, the urinary bladder, and the uterus.

HISTOLOGIC STRUCTURE OF THE MUCOUS MEMBRANES

Histologically, a mucous membrane is a modified skin. It is made of two layers: a surface layer of *epithelial tissue* and an underlying layer of *connective tissue* (called *lamina propria*). Mucous membranes are structurally less thick and tough than the skin. Whereas the skin is kept slightly moist by secretions from oil and sweat glands that empty onto the surface, mucous membranes are kept moist by secretions from mucous and serous glands or other secretory cells that empty onto the surface. The epithelium of a mucous membrane is primarily protective in function, but in some areas it is also secretory and absorptive in function. The connective tissue of a mucous membrane underlies the epithelium and contains blood vessels, nerves, and sometimes glands.

Mucous membranes in different parts of the body differ in several ways, and, in each location, their structure appears to be excellently suited to the functions they perform. Mucous membranes that are normally protected from wear and tear are thin and delicate, but mucous membranes that are subject to functional friction are thicker and resistant to injury.

Protected cavities, such as the nasal cavity, the stomach, and the intestines, are lined by delicate types of mucous membranes. In the nasal cavity, the epithelial part of the mucous membrane is composed of pseudostratified columnar cells (see Fig. 1-3D). Many of these columnar cells have cilia—tiny, hair-like projections—on their exposed ends; other cells called *goblet cells* secrete mucus,[1] which keeps the surface of the mucosa moist. The connective tissue part of the nasal mucous membrane is likewise thin and delicate and contains nerves, blood vessels, mucous, and serous glands that open onto the surface of the mucosa. This moist, ciliated mu-

---

[1] *Mucus* (noun) is a viscous, watery secretion that covers a *mucous* (adjective) membrane. *Mucosa* (noun) is another name for mucous membrane.

cous membrane of the nasal passage functions as a dirt-catcher and helps to prevent dust inhaled with air from reaching the lungs.

Lining the stomach is a mucous membrane that is somewhat thicker than that of the nasal cavity and is arranged in many folds and wrinkles. The epithelium of the stomach mucosa is made of simple columnar cells that are without cilia and have a secretory function (see Fig. 1-3C). The underlying connective tissue contains many glands.

The mucosa of the small intestine resembles the stomach mucosa in many respects. It has an epithelium composed of simple columnar cells; some of these cells are goblet cells that secrete mucus, and others absorb food materials from the intestine. The connective tissue contains many glands.

In contrast to the protected, delicate mucous membranes of the nasal cavity, the stomach, and the intestines, the mucosa that lines the oral cavity is sturdier. The lining of the mouth is constantly subject to rubbing and scraping by the process of mastication of food as well as by the presence of the teeth in the mouth. As in other areas, the structure of the mucous membrane of the oral cavity is suited to its usage.

ORAL MUCOUS MEMBRANE

Histologic Structure of the Oral Mucous Membrane

The mucous membrane that lines the mouth is heavier and more resistant to injury than are the mucous membranes of more protected cavities. The histologic structure of the *oral mucosa* enables it to withstand the wear and tear of ordinary oral function and to resist bacterial infection. Like all mucous membranes, the oral mucosa is composed of a combination of epithelial and connective tissues (Fig. 10-1). The surface epithelial tissue is attached to the underlying connective tissue by a basement membrane (see Fig. 1-3).

The epithelial portion of the oral mucosa is *stratified squamous* in character; that is, the epithelial cells are mostly flat and are several layers deep (see Fig. 1-3E). As in all stratified squamous epithelium, the basal layer of epithelial cells, which rests upon the connective tissue, is composed of cuboidal rather than flat cells. Most of the cell division takes place in this basal layer. As new epithelial cells are produced by mitosis in the basal layer, some basal cells and cells superficial to them are forced outward and eventually reach the surface.

Different things happen to these surface epithelial cells in different parts of the mouth. In areas of the mouth in which the mucosa is relatively protected, such as on the inside of the cheeks and lips and on the underside of the tongue, the surface epithelial cells are sloughed off into the saliva as new epithelial cells are produced in the basal layer. If a scraping from the inside of the cheeks is spread onto a glass slide and examined under a microscope, squamous epithelial cells will be visible.

In parts of the mouth in which the oral mucosa is subject to considerable wear and tear, such as the hard palate and gingiva, the surface epithelial cells are not sloughed off. Instead, they lose their nuclei and cell boundaries and form a noncellular, tough, protective layer on the surface of the stratified squamous epithelial cells. This tough layer is called the *keratin layer*, and the epithelium upon which

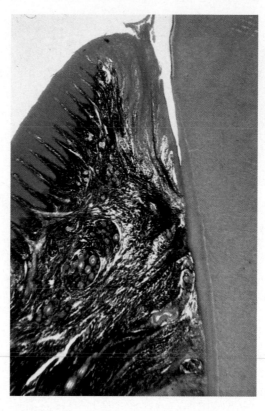

Figure 10–1. (See Color Plates) Microscopic view of free gingiva adjacent to the cervical part of a tooth. Notice the interdigitation of the surface epithelium with the underlying fibrous connective tissue (lamina propria) and the attachment of the fibers to the cementum.

such a layer occurs is called *keratinized*[2] *epithelium* (Figs.10-2 and 10-3). The keratin layer wears with use but is continuously replaced by the younger cells beneath it.

The connective tissue portion of the oral mucosa is chiefly composed of fibrous connective tissue that contains blood vessels and nerves. It is separated from the overlying stratified squamous epithelium by a thin basement membrane. In most places, the boundary between the connective tissue and epithelium is irregular and contains projections of connective tissue that extend like fingers into the epithelium but do not reach the surface. In some areas of the oral mucosa, these projections are characteristically much longer and numerous than in other areas (Figs. 10-1 and 10-3). The irregularity of contact surfaces between the tissues serves to increase the area from which the epithelium can receive nourishment from the underlying connective tissue.

The connective tissue of the oral mucosa varies both in thickness in different parts of the mouth and in the nature of its attachment to the underlying tissue. In some areas of the mouth, the connective tissue of the oral mucosa is attached firmly to underlying bone, as in the part of the gingiva that is attached to the periosteum of the alveolar process. In other areas, the connective tissue of the oral mucosa rests upon a looser type of connective tissue called the *submucosa*, which contains larger blood vessels, nerves, glands, and fat tissue. Such an attachment of

---

[2]Pronounced *kĕr′ a tĭn īzed.*

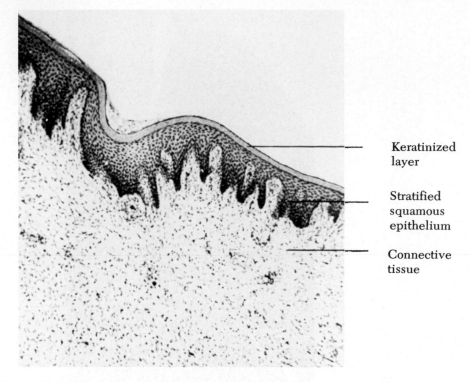

Keratinized
layer

Stratified
squamous
epithelium

Connective
tissue

Figure 10–2. Photomicrograph of a section of human gingiva, low-power magnification.

oral mucosa to submucosa is seen in the cheek. The character of the submucosa varies in different parts of the mouth, and its nature helps to determine the character of the mucosa that it supports.

For convenience of discussion, an attempt has been made to classify the different areas of oral mucosa. The classification divides the oral mucosa into three categories: masticatory mucosa, lining mucosa, and specialized mucosa. If you carefully examine someone's mouth and observe the mucosa in different places, such a division will seem logical.

Masticatory mucosa
    Gingiva
    Hard palate
Lining mucosa
    Lips and cheeks
    Floor of mouth
    Underside of tongue
    Soft palate
    Alveolar mucosa
Specialized mucosa
    Dorsum of tongue

Masticatory mucosa is the name given to the mucous membrane of the *gingiva* and *hard palate*. These areas of the oral mucosa are most used during the mastication of food. The epithelium of the masticatory mucosa is usually keratinized.

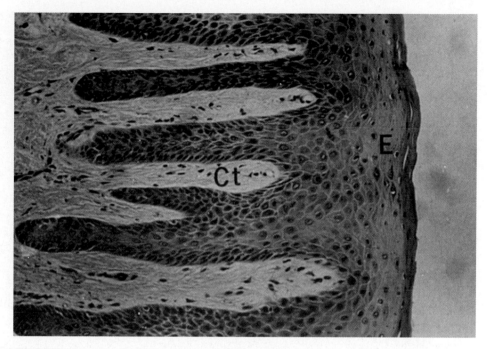

Figure 10–3. Higher magnification of the gingival epithelial (E) and connective tissue (CT) layers. Clearly seen are the stratified arrangement of epithelial cells and the interdigitation of the epithelium and connective tissue. The surface layer of the epithelium is keratin.

By looking into a person's mouth, you can see that the necks of the teeth and the bone in which the teeth are set are covered with a firm mucous membrane that fits closely around the teeth and is tightly attached to the bone. This part of the oral mucosa is called gingiva (Figs. 10-4 and 10-5). The firm gingiva is usually keratinized and has a stippled appearance. Except for a narrow zone around the necks of the teeth, the gingival mucosa is attached firmly to the underlying tissue. Examining the facial side of the upper and lower jaws reveals that, several millimeters rootward from the margin of the gingiva, a scalloped line divides the gingival mucosa from the alveolar mucosa (Figs. 10-4 and 10-5). The *alveolar mucosa* may be distinguished from gingiva because it is redder, shiny, and loose fitting. Figure 10-6 clearly shows the scalloped junction between the gingival and alveolar mucosae.

The mucosa that covers the hard palate is usually well keratinized (Fig. 10-7). It is attached directly to the bone of the roof of the mouth only in the area of the *palatine raphe*,[3] which is the anteroposterior elevation in the center of the hard palate that you can feel with your tongue. On either side of the palatine raphe, a submucosa separates the palatine mucosa from the bone. The submucosa in the anterior part of the hard palate contains much fat tissue and in the posterior part contains large salivary glands of the mucous type. The ducts of these glands open onto the surface of the palate mucosa, but these small openings usually are not visible to the naked eye.

---

[3] Pronounced *rā′ fē* (fr. Greek *raphe* = a seam or suture).

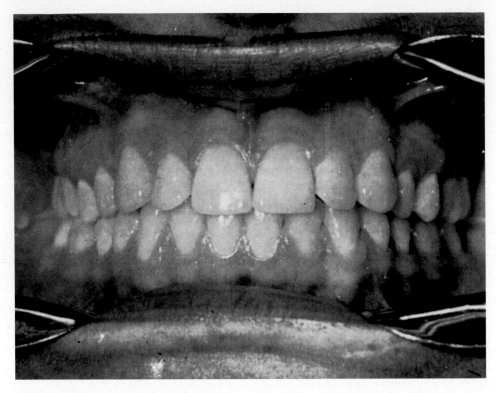

Figure 10–4. The subject of this photograph was a 22-year-old woman. The gingival margin fits snugly against the enamel of the tooth crowns, and the interdental papillae fill the interdental spaces (i.e., the space between the teeth cervical to the areas of contact). The alveolar mucosa is clearly seen in the maxillary vestibule and less clearly in the mandibular vestibule.

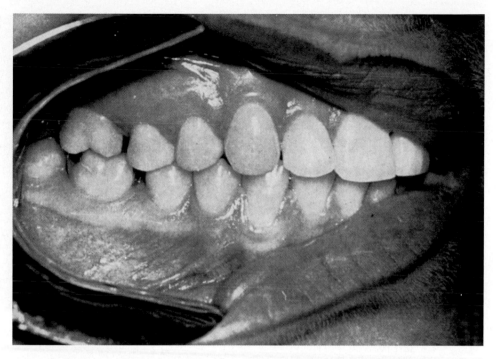

Figure 10–5. The subject is the same as that in Fig. 10-4. The line between the gingiva and alveolar mucosa of the lower jaw is clear. Notice the loose-fitting appearance of the alveolar mucosa and the minute blood vessels that are close to the surface. The firm gingiva is light in color and has a stippled (pitted) surface texture.

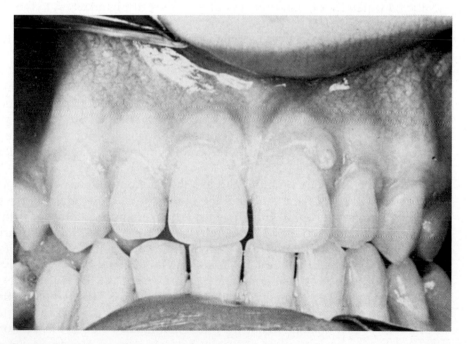

Figure 10–6. This subject has a clear scalloped line between the gingiva (masticatory mucosa) and the alveolar mucosa (lining mucosa) in the upper facial area. On close inspection, small blood vessels are seen in the thinner, nonkeratinized alveolar mucosa.

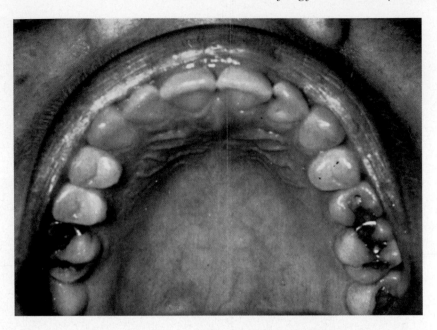

Figure 10–7. The subject is the same as that in Fig. 10-4. The hard palate is well keratinized; the palatine rugae[4] (horizontal ridges behind the anterior teeth) are distinct. The palatine raphe, distinguished with difficulty in this photograph, extends from anterior to posterior in the center line. Notice how the gingiva fits snugly around the palatal sides of the teeth.

Notwithstanding the presence of the fat and gland tissue in the submucosa of the hard palate, the oral mucosa in this area is firmly attached to the underlying bone structure. This attachment is accomplished by strands of connective tissue that extend from the mucosa through the submucosa and attach firmly to the bone of the roof of the mouth.

Lining mucosa is located in areas of the oral cavity in which the mucous membrane may logically be thought to function as a lining rather than as a masticatory organ. Such nonmasticatory areas are the floor of the mouth and the underside of the tongue (Fig. 10-8), the alveolar mucosa (Fig. 10-6), the soft palate, and the inside of the cheeks and lips. In none of these areas is the mucosa firmly attached to underlying bone, and ordinarily the epithelium in these areas is not keratinized (Fig. 10-9).

Examine someone's mouth, and ask the person to lift his or her tongue (Fig. 10-8). The floor of the mouth and the underside of the tongue are covered with lining mucosa, the epithelium of which is nonkeratinized, shiny, and thin enough that blood vessels located in the underlying connective tissue are clearly visible. The fold of mucosa that extends lengthwise in the center of the undersurface of the tongue is the *lingual frenum*. Comparing this frenum in several individuals reveals that it varies considerably in size and extent. At the lower end of the lingual frenum, where the undersurface of the tongue is attached to the floor of the mouth, a nearly horizontal fold of tissue extends to the right and left of the frenum. This horizontal fold is the plica sublingualis.[5] Along the crest of the plica

---

[4]Plural, pronounced *rū′ ge;* singular is *ruga,* pronounced *rōō′ gȧ.*
[5]Pronounced *pli′ kȧ süb lĭng guăl ĭs.*

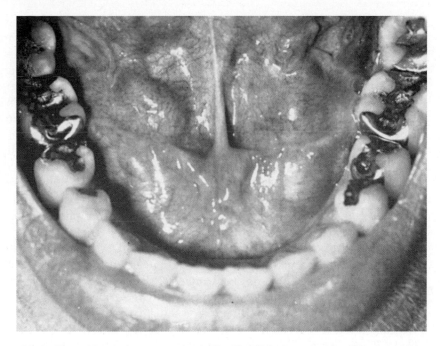

Figure 10–8. The subject is the same as that in Fig. 10-4. This photograph is of the floor of the mouth and part of the undersurface of the elevated tongue. The mandibular anterior teeth are at the bottom of the picture. The lingual frenum, which holds the tongue to the floor of the mouth, divides the area into right and left halves. The horizontal fold—the sublingual fold or plica sublingualis—that extends from the base of the tongue to the floor of the mouth bears the openings of the ducts from the sublingual and submandibular glands.

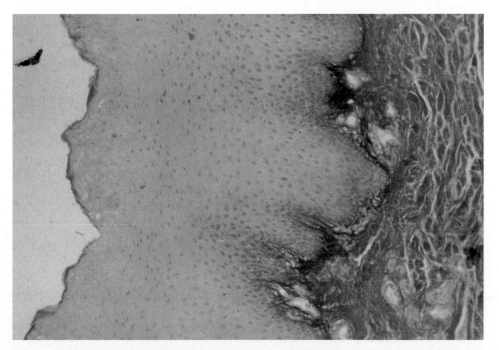

Figure 10–9. (See Color Plates) Microscopic view of a section of cheek mucosa. Notice the thick epithelial layer and the lack of both a keratin surface layer and the interdigitation of the epithelium and connective tissue. Compare this lining type of oral mucosa to the masticatory type seen in Fig. 10-3.

sublingualis are small openings of ducts that are usually not visible to the naked eye; these ducts lead from the sublingual salivary glands and empty into the mouth beneath the tongue. In the center of the plica sublingualis, the larger openings of *Wharton's ducts*, one on either side of the base of the lingual frenum, carry the salivary secretions from the submandibular and sublingual glands to the oral cavity. If you have ever opened your mouth and been surprised by two thin streams of saliva shooting out from beneath your tongue, you now know where they came from.

Now, continuing your examination of the mouth, pull the lower lip down and out and the upper lip up and out; then, pull the cheeks back at the corners of the mouth. Notice the alveolar mucosa that lines the oral vestibules.[6] The epithelium of this mucosa is nonkeratinized, shiny, red, and partially transparent to underlying blood vessels. It is clearly demarcated from the paler gingiva mucosa by a scalloped line (Figs. 10-5 and 10-6).

The *soft palate*, which begins distal to the maxillary third molar teeth, is a mass of flexible muscle covered on the oral surface with oral mucosa. The epithelium of this mucosa ordinarily is not keratinized. Numerous salivary glands lie beneath the mucosa of the soft palate and empty onto its surface.

Examining the cheek mucosa inside the corners of the mouth of several individuals often reveals an area that contains small, yellowish spots called *Fordyce's spots*. These spots are openings onto the oral mucosa of sebaceous glands, which usually are thought to be restricted to the skin on the outside of the body. It is believed that they occur in this area as a result of the narrowing of the wide embryonic mouth during early facial development. In other words, during the filling in of the angle between the maxillary process and mandibular arch at either corner of the mouth, some skin glands become entrapped. However near fact this explanation may be, it does not account for the presence of sebaceous glands on the red margin of the upper lip; their usual absence on the lower lip; their presence on areas of cheek mucosa above, below, and behind the area of narrowing of the embryonic mouth; their seeming absence in human fetuses; nor their greater number in adults than in children.

Specialized mucosa is the term applied to the mucous membrane located on the dorsum (top side) of the tongue. The mucosa in this area is distinctly different from other oral mucosa. By examining someone's tongue, you can see that the mucosa of its upper surface is formed into innumerable small hills or *papillae*. These papillae vary in type, size, and shape, and some of them bear microscopic organs that supply the sense of taste.

Filiform papillae (Figs. 10-10, 10-11, and 10-12) are thread-like in appearance, cover the top surface of the tongue, and give it a velvety appearance. The epithelium that covers the tips of filiform papillae is usually heavily keratinized (Fig. 10-13). In the human tongue, the keratinization is not sufficient to impart the sandpaper-like quality of the keratinized papillae on a kitten's tongue.

Fungiform papillae (Figs. 10-10 and 10-14) are mushroom-shaped, larger, and less numerous than filiform papillae. They are scattered among but because of their

---

[6] The maxillary and mandibular *oral vestibules* are the spaces between the facial surfaces of the teeth and their supporting bone and the oral surfaces of the cheeks and lips. A finger that is inserted into the mouth between the teeth and the cheek or lip is in the *vestibule*.

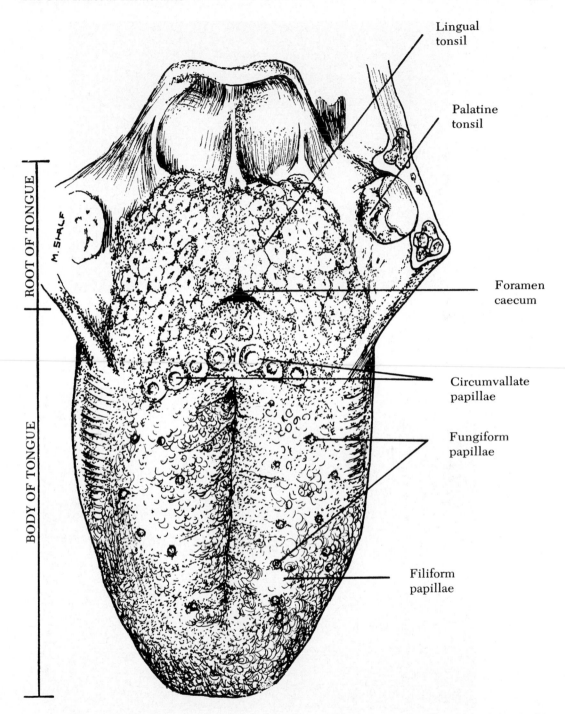

Figure 10–10. Diagrammatic drawing of the dorsum of the human tongue. The division between the body and root is indicated, as are the locations of papillae types, the foramen cecum, and the lingual tonsil.

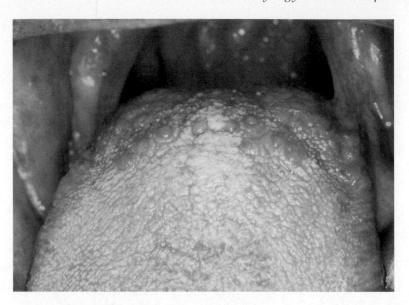

Figure 10–11. (See Color Plates) Clinical view of the dorsum of the posterior or root of the tongue. Note the large prominent circumvallate papillae arranged in a V pattern. Can you locate the three other types of lingual papillae? See the labels in Fig. 10-10.

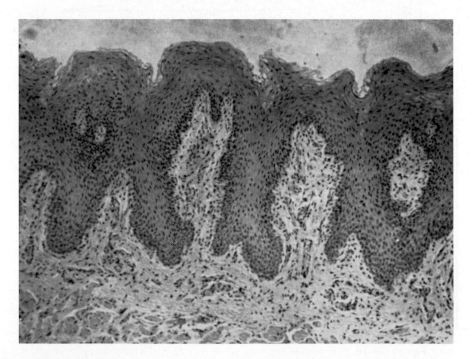

Figure 10–12. Photomicrograph of a vertical section through the upper surface of a human tongue. These are filiform papillae. In this section, the surface of the epithelium does not appear to be heavily keratinized.

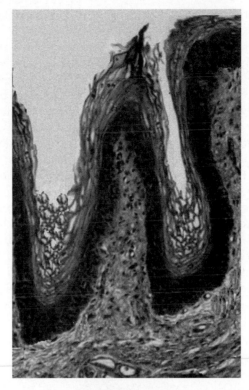

Figure 10–13. Histologic section of a filiform papilla showing heavy keratinization. The dark area is the rest of the epithelium. Notice the core of connective tissue underlying the epithelium.

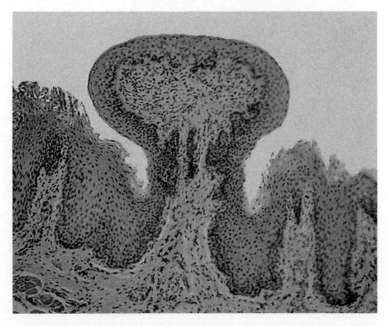

Figure 10–14. Photomicrograph of a vertical section through the upper surface of a human tongue demonstrates a fungiform papilla. Examine someone's tongue, and locate some papillae of this type.

thinner epithelium appear redder than filiform papillae. They may be clearly seen by careful examination of the tongue.

Foliate papillae are located along the lateral borders of the posterior part of the tongue. In the human tongue, these papillae are not well developed (Fig. 10-15).

Circumvallate papillae (Figs. 10-10, 10-11, and 10-15), which are also called *vallate papillae*, are located well back on the tongue, between its body and base. These relatively large, conspicuous structures number from eight to 10 and are arranged in a V-shaped line, with the point of the V directed toward the throat. Each papilla is surrounded by a trench, or trough, into the bottom of which open ducts that lead from the salivary or *von Ebner's* glands located beneath them. The saliva from these glands floods the trench around the papilla and serves as a solvent for food substances.

Along the lateral surfaces of these papillae are groups of specialized epithelial cells called *taste buds*. When food substances that are in solution in the saliva from von Ebner's glands come in contact with taste buds, an individual experiences a sensation of taste.

Fungiform, foliate, and circumvallate papillae all contain organs of taste, but they are more conspicuous on the circumvallate papillae.

Figure 10-16 is a photomicrograph of a section of rabbit tongue in the area of the

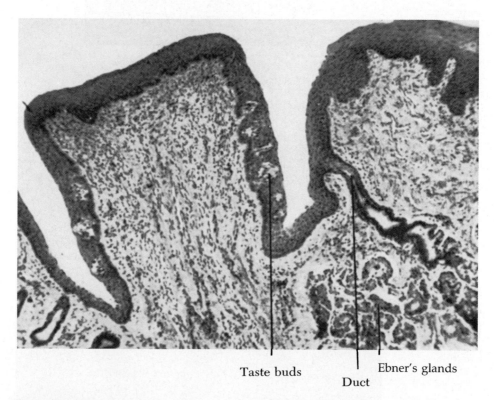

Taste buds   Ebner's glands
Duct

Figure 10–15. Photomicrograph of a vertical section through the dorsum (upper surface) of a human tongue demonstrates a circumvallate papilla. The papillae may 2–3 mm in diameter. Taste buds are located along the side surface; a duct from von Ebner's salivary glands empties into the base of the trench around the papilla. This section is cut through the length of the duct, just to one side of the duct opening. Consequently, the exact point at which the duct opens into the trench cannot be seen.

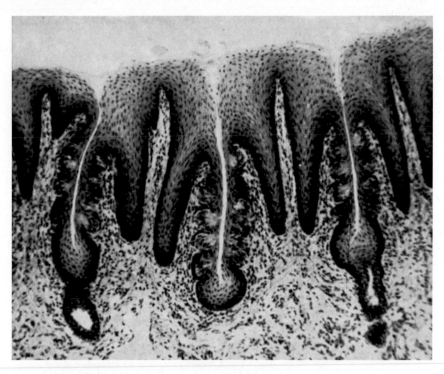

Figure 10–16. Photomicrograph of a section through the side of a rabbit tongue. These foliate papillae are shaped differently but are better developed in a rabbit than in a human. The taste buds are clearly seen in the epithelium along the sides of the papillae. See Fig. 10-17 for an enlargement.

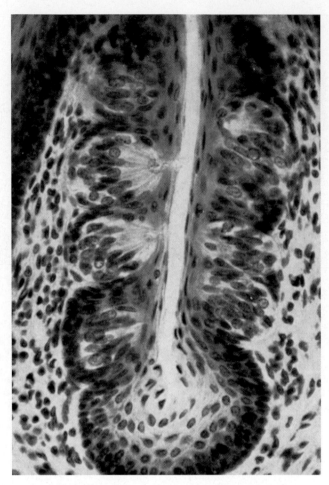

Figure 10–17. Photomicrograph at a higher magnification of the taste buds seen in the center of the picture in Fig. 10-16. On the left of the vertical space between the two papillae, two taste buds are cut through their centers. Notice the pore-like opening to the surface.

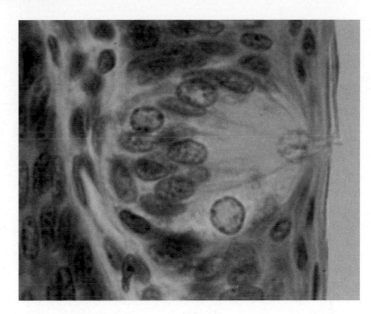

Figure 10–18. (See Color Plates) Highly magnified view of a taste bud. Note that the taste cells of the bud are arranged like the staves of a barrel and that their nuclei (left) are at the base, opposite to the position of the taste pore at the surface (right).

foliate papillae. Note the taste buds along the sides of the papillae. Although these rabbit papillae are shaped differently than human circumvallate papillae, they are more easily studied in the rabbit tongue. Figure 10-17 is a higher magnification of the taste buds seen in the center of Figure 10-16. Notice the fine detail of their construction in Figure 10-18. The taste pore, which allows food substances access to the taste receptor cells, is at the right and contains small cilia that protrude through the overlying ectoderm.

SELECTED READINGS

Long RG, Hlousek L, Doyle JL. Oral manifestations of systemic diseases. Mt Sinai J Med 1998;65:309–315.

MacPhail LA, Greenspan JS. Oral ulceration in HIV infection: investigation and pathogenesis. Oral Diseases 1997;3 Suppl 1:S190–S193.

Myers J, Squire CA, Gerson SJ. The Structure and Function of Oral Mucosa. New York: Pergemon Press; 1984.

Porter SR, Scully C, Pedersen A. Recurrent aphthous stomatitis. Crit Rev Oral Biol Med;9:306–321.

Spijkervet FK, Sonis ST. New frontiers in the management of chemotherapy-induced mucositis. Curr Opin Oncol;10 Suppl 1:S23–S27.

11 The Gingiva

LOCATION

Gingiva is the part of the oral mucosa that surrounds the cervices of the teeth; it is firmly attached to the alveolar process and the cervical parts of the teeth. Gingiva on the facial side of the maxillae and mandible in the premolar and molar regions is called *buccal gingiva*; in the incisor and canine regions, it is called *labial gingiva*. Gingiva on the inside of the mandibular arch is called *lingual gingiva*; on the inside of the maxillary arch, it is called *palatal gingiva*.

CLINICAL APPEARANCE

The clinical appearance of the gingiva can be studied by examining your own mouth or that of a classmate. Pull the lower lip out and down and the upper lip out and up. Below the crowns of the mandibular teeth and above the crowns of the maxillary teeth, the oral mucous membrane is firm and has a stippled, or finely pitted, surface. This membrane is gingiva. In people who have fair skin, the color of the gingiva is a slightly grayish pink. In dark-complexioned individuals, the gingiva frequently either is spotted with brown or is a fairly even grayish brown as a result of the melanin found in some epithelial cells. Around the facial surface of the anterior teeth, 4 or 5 mm from the cervical margin, the gingiva ends in a scalloped line. The oral mucosa beyond this line is red, shiny, and loosely attached to the underlying tissue (Fig. 11-1). Examine also the gingiva around the buccal side of the mandibular and maxillary posterior teeth. The color and surface textures here are the same as those in the anterior region, and a scalloped line marks the apical border.

Now examine the lingual side of the mandibular arch. The gingiva is firmly attached to the hard underlying tissue, whereas oral mucosa beneath the tongue is loose, shiny, and redder in color than the gingiva. Examine the palatal side of the maxillary arch. On the maxilla, the palatal gingiva blends without a distinct line into the oral mucosa of the hard palate (Fig. 11-2).

Look again at the facial, lingual, and palatal surfaces of the mandibular and maxillary arches. The position and shape of the gingival margin depend largely on the age of the individual. In a young person, the gingiva covers the cervical part of the enamel of the tooth, such that the *clinical crown* (the part of the tooth exposed in the oral cavity) is smaller than the *anatomic crown* (the part of the tooth that has an enamel surface). Between the teeth, a triangular wedge of gingiva, the *interdental papilla*, fills the interproximal space (Fig. 11-1).

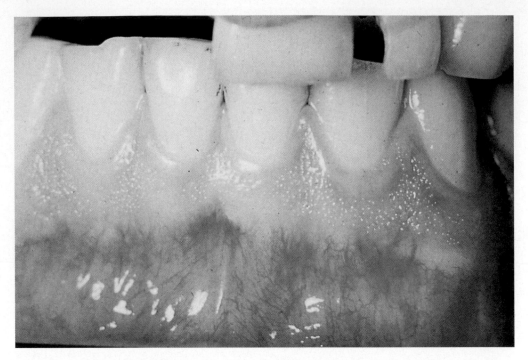

Figure 11–1. (See Color Plates) Facial side of the anterior mandibular arch. The line between the gingiva and alveolar mucosa is clear. The gingiva is firm, light in color, and stippled in appearance; the interdental papilla fills the interproximal spaces; and the gingival margin can still be observed on the enamel of all teeth. Minute blood vessels are clearly seen in the red, shiny alveolar mucosa.

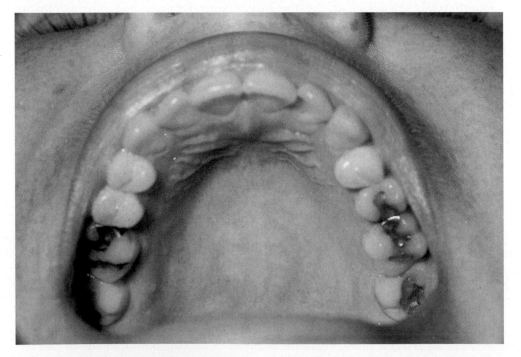

Figure 11–2. (See Color Plates) Palatal surface of the maxillary arch. The palatal gingiva blends with the mucosa of the hard palate without a line of demarcation. An alveolar mucosa is not present in this area.

Between the teeth, where the interdental papilla meets or nearly meets the point of tooth contact, an indentation, or depression, is seen on the crest of the papilla. This depression is called a col[1] and may be a sheltered reservoir for entrapped food. When adjacent teeth do not touch, or when a tooth is missing, the interdental papilla and col are not present.

In a person 30 or 35 years of age, the interdental papillae may not extend to the areas of tooth contact, and most or all of the tooth enamel is most likely uncovered. In such cases, the clinical and anatomic crowns are often approximately the same.

Now examine a person 50 or 60 years old, and compare your findings with those in the young person and younger adult. In the middle-aged or older person, not only do the interdental papillae often fail to fill the spaces that exist between the teeth cervical to the contact areas (the interproximal spaces); on some or all surfaces of the teeth, cementum often can also be seen around the cervix (Fig. 11-3). The gingival margin in such an older person is located so far rootward that some of the root cementum is exposed in the oral cavity, and the clinical crown of the tooth is larger than the anatomic crown.

This age-related change in the position of the gingiva on the tooth is expected to occur, just as hair is expected to become gray and skin to become wrinkled with age. However, at any age, diseases of the tissues around the teeth may produce pathologic changes that result in gingival recession. This review discusses usual and expected age-related changes.

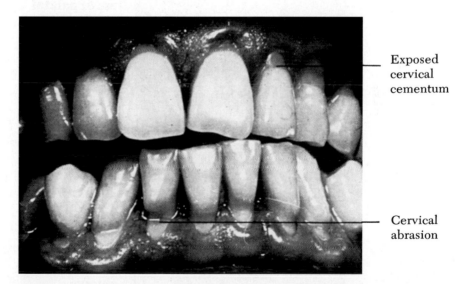

Exposed cervical cementum

Cervical abrasion

Figure 11–3. Clinical photograph of maxillary and mandibular anterior teeth with associated gingiva. The subject was 60 years old. Notice the stippled gingiva, the position of the interdental papillae, and the exposed but undamaged cementum on the left maxillary lateral incisor and on the right maxillary central incisor. The exposed and deeply cut cementum on the mandibular anterior teeth is cervical abrasion.

---

[1] Pronounced *kôl*. The word *col* usually refers to a pass between adjacent peaks of a mountain chain. In this case, the facial and lingual points of the interdental papilla represent the adjacent mountain peaks, and the depression between them is the col.

HISTOLOGIC STRUCTURE

Gingiva is a masticatory type of oral mucous membrane (see Chapter 10). Like other areas of the oral mucous membrane, the gingiva is composed of both connective and epithelial tissues (Fig. 11-4). The connective tissue (called *lamina propria*) is of the fibrous type, whereas the surface epithelial tissue is stratified squamous in character and usually keratinized (see Fig. 10-2). This keratinization causes the color of the gingiva to be grayish pink, rather than red if it is not pigmented, or grayish brown, rather than reddish brown if pigmentation is present. The finger-shaped projections of the connective tissue that extend into the epithelium (Fig. 11-5) most likely produce the pitted condition of the surface of the epithelium in some areas. The gingiva does not have a submucosa, but rests directly on the underlying hard tissue. Ordinarily, the gingiva contains no salivary glands (Fig. 11-6).

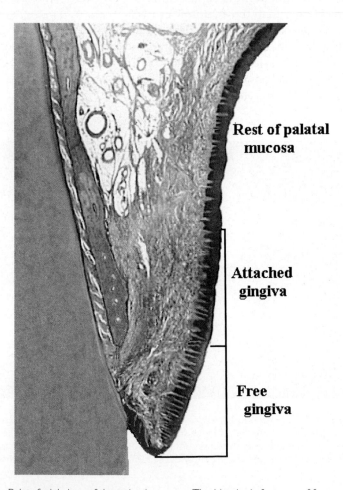

Figure 11–4. Palatofacial view of the palatal mucosa. The histologic features of free and attached gingiva and their relation to the alveolar bone and root of the tooth (left) are shown. The clear area (top) within the palatal mucosa is a submucosa that contains palatine blood vessels and nerves. Can you locate the periodontal ligament?

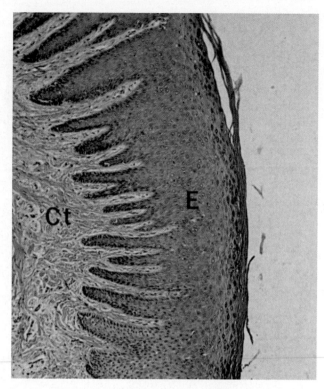

Figure 11–5. Section of human gingiva showing the interdigitation between the keratinized stratified squamous epithelium (E) and the fibrous connective tissue (CT). A portion of the keratin (above) has pulled away from the adjacent epithelial cells.

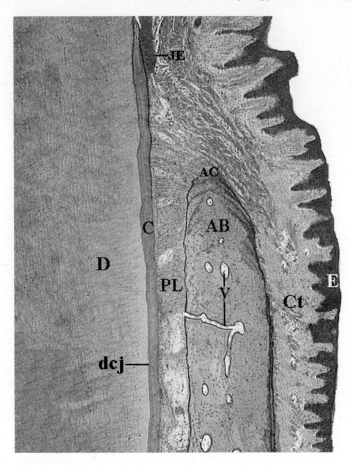

Figure 11–6. (See Color Plates) Histologic section through a portion of the gingiva and its underlying structures. E, epithelium of the gingiva; CT, connective tissue or lamina propria of the gingiva; AB, alveolar bone; AC, crest of alveolar bone; V, enclosed vascular canals of alveolar bone; PL, periodontal ligament; C, cementum; D, dentin; DCJ, dentinocemental junction; JE, junctional epithelial attachment to the cementum.

The connective tissue of the free gingiva contains several particularly oriented sets of collagen fibers (Figs. 11-7 and 11-8). The groups of periodontal ligament fibers that penetrate the lamina propria of the gingiva are the transseptal fibers and the free gingival or dentogingival fibers (Fig. 11-7; see Fig. 8-1). The transseptal fibers pass from the cementum of one tooth, over the crest of the interdental bone, to the cementum of another tooth; they are confined to the area between teeth. Free gingival fibers pass from the cementum to the lamina propria of the free gingiva; they are located on all sides of a tooth.

Three other groups of fibers are also located in the connective tissue of the gingiva. The dentoperiosteal fibers pass from the cervical cementum to the facial and lingual cortical bone surfaces of the alveolar process; they are confined to the facial and lingual sides of a tooth (Fig 11-8). The alveologingival fibers pass from the crest of the alveolar bone to the lamina propria of the free gingiva; they surround the entire tooth (Fig. 11-9). The circular fibers are attached neither to cementum nor to bone; they encircle the tooth like a ring (Fig. 11-10).

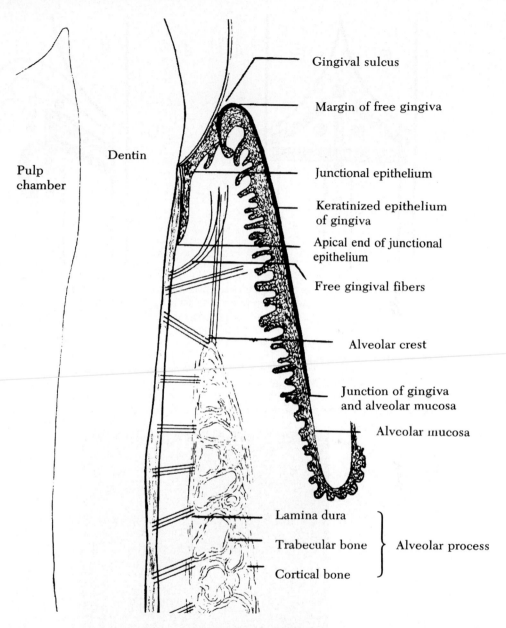

Pulp chamber

Dentin

Gingival sulcus

Margin of free gingiva

Junctional epithelium

Keratinized epithelium of gingiva

Apical end of junctional epithelium

Free gingival fibers

Alveolar crest

Junction of gingiva and alveolar mucosa

Alveolar mucosa

Lamina dura

Trabecular bone

Cortical bone

Alveolar process

Figure 11–7. Diagrammatic drawing of a section of the buccal cervical area of a mandibular molar, cut buccolingually.

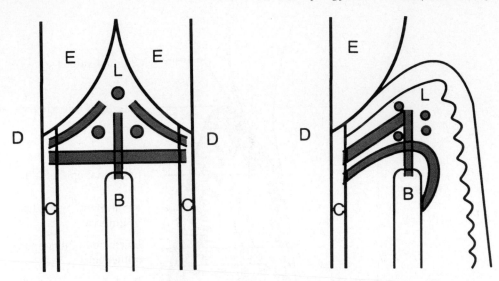

Figure 11–8. Diagram of the functionally arranged fibers within the lamina propria (L) of the free gingiva. The interdental papilla fibers are illustrated (left): dentinogingival fibers extend from the cementum (C) of adjacent teeth and pass into the lamina propria; transseptal fibers extend from the cementum of one tooth, pass over the crest of the interdental bone (B), and continue to the cementum of the other tooth; alveologingival fibers pass from the crest of the alveolar bone to the lamina propria; and circular fibers lie free in the lamina propria. The arrangement of the gingival fibers (right) as seen on the facial or lingual side of a tooth are also illustrated (right): dentinogingival fibers pass from the cementum (C) to the lamina propria (L); dentinoperiosteal fibers extend from the cementum and pass over the alveolar bone (B) crest to the cortical plate; alveologingival fibers pass from the bone crest to the lamina propria; and circular fibers are free in the lamina propria. E, enamel; D, dentin.

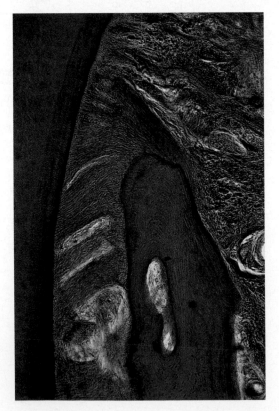

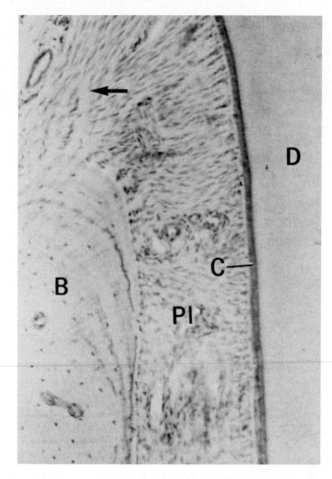

Figure 11–10. Microscopic view of the bone crest (B) area of the alveolar process. The alveologingival fibers (arrow) of the gingiva pass from within the alveolar bone crest to the connective tissue of the gingiva. The epithelium of the gingiva is above the area of this figure. PL, periodontal ligament; C, cementum; D, dentin.

Figure 11–9. (See Color Plates) Faciolingual histologic section of the mandibular crest region. Note the prominent dentinoperiosteal fibers of the gingiva that pass from the cervical area of the tooth (left), over the crest of the alveolar bone, to the periosteum of the mandibular cortical bone. Dentinogingival and circular fibers are seen above the dentinoperiosteal fibers. Notice the arrangement of periodontal ligament fibers. The section was specially prepared to reveal fibers; cells are not seen.

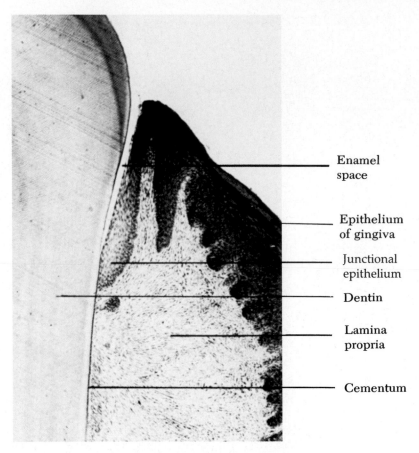

Figure 11-11. Section of a tooth and its associated gingiva. The junctional epithelium is adjacent to the enamel and cementum of the tooth. The enamel space is observed where the enamel had been before the tooth was demineralized; the enamel was lost during the demineralization process. (See Chapter 1.)

THE GINGIVAL SULCUS

Beneath the coronal border of the gingiva in all teeth is a space, or crevice, called the *gingival sulcus* (Fig. 11-7). A small dental instrument can be inserted into this space as far as the bottom of the gingival sulcus. This border of the gingiva that is not attached to the tooth surface is called the *free gingiva*. The inner wall of the sulcus is, of course, the tooth surface. The outer wall is the stratified squamous epithelium of the gingival sulcus, which is continuous coronally over the *gingival margin* with the stratified squamous epithelium of the outer surface of the gingiva; apically, the outer wall is continuous with the *junctional epithelium* (Figs. 11-7 and 11-11).

The depth of the gingival sulcus has been reported to vary from 0 to 6 mm. The preferable depth is usually considered to be near 0 mm. The depth of the sulcus is marked on the surface of the gingiva by a horizontal depression called the *free gingival groove*.

THE JUNCTIONAL EPITHELIUM

The junctional epithelium (also called *attachment epithelium*) is the band of stratified squamous epithelium that is attached to the tooth surface around the cervical part of all teeth. It is continuous coronally with the epithelium of the gingival sulcus and over the gingival margin with the epithelium on the outer surface of the gingiva (Figs. 11-7, 11-11, 11-12, and 11-13).

The epithelial cells of the junctional epithelium that lie adjacent to the tooth surface produce a structure that resembles the basal lamina of a basement membrane (see Chapter 1). This structure is the attaching substance between the cells of the junctional epithelium and the tooth.

In young individuals, the junctional epithelium ends apically at the cemento-enamel junction (Figs. 11-7 and 11-14). At this early stage of tooth eruption, the clinical crown is short because the cervical part of the enamel is covered with gingiva. As tooth eruption continues, the gingiva recedes cervically, thus exposing more of the anatomic crown. At the same time, the apical end of the junctional epithelium slowly migrates and grows by cell division onto the cementum in the cervical part of the root. It becomes firmly attached to the cementum (Fig. 11-13).

With age, the gingiva continues slowly to move rootward from the crown of the tooth, and the junctional epithelium continues slowly to grow apically on the cementum. This process is in part a consequence of the slow occlusal tooth movement that appears to occur, most likely intermittently, throughout the life of the

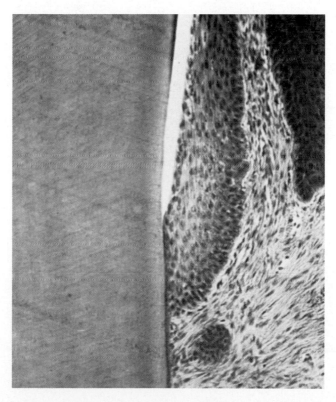

Figure 11–12. Higher magnification of the junctional epithelium seen in Fig. 11-11. The close association of the junctional epithelium to the tooth surface is clear, as is its stratified cellular arrangement.

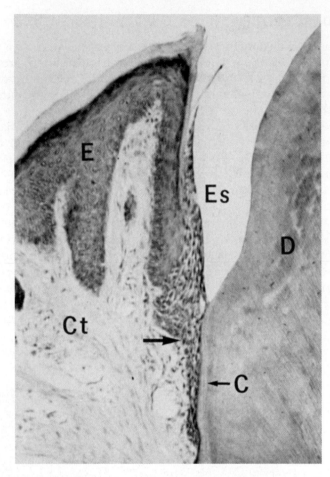

Figure 11–13. Histologic section of the dentinogingival area. The junctional epithelium (arrow) extends from its attachment to the enamel (ES) to its attachment to the cementum (C). The junctional epithelium is continuous with the gingival epithelium (E) and is attached to the connective tissue (CT) of the gingiva. The enamel space (ES) is the area occupied by enamel prior to demineralization. Notice the thick keratin layer at the surface of the gingiva. D, dentin.

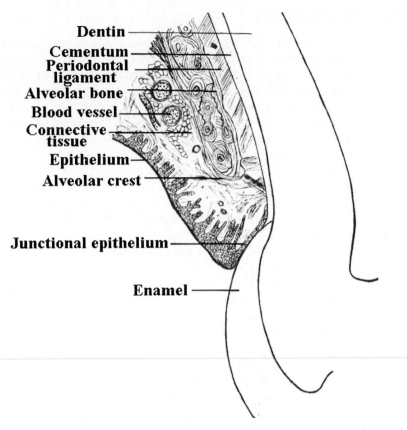

Dentin

Cementum

Periodontal ligament

Alveolar bone

Blood vessel

Connective tissue

Epithelium

Alveolar crest

Junctional epithelium

Enamel

Figure 11–14. Diagrammatic drawing of a longitudinal section through a maxillary posterior tooth and the associated periodontal ligament, alveolar process, and gingiva; cut faciolingually. This illustration demonstrates the lingual side of the tooth at the cervix. This area is free of inflammation, and bone resorption is not observed. The periodontal ligament fibers are well oriented.

tooth. Chiefly, however, this apical growth of epithelium appears to occur independently of occlusal tooth movement and is referred to as the *rootward migration of the junctional epithelium*. This aging process is natural and therefore not accompanied by inflammation. As aging continues, the gingiva recedes to the extent that the tooth crown becomes completely uncovered and exposed to the oral cavity. Afterward, continued gingival recession exposes cervical cementum and places the junctional epithelium considerably apical to the cementoenamel junction (Fig. 11-3). When the cementum is exposed, the bottom of the gingival sulcus is, of course, somewhere on the tooth root; however, it is not necessarily found at the same level on all the teeth in a mouth, nor is it even on all sides of the same tooth. In a healthy mouth, the gingival sulcus under these conditions is ordinarily shallow.

Exposure of cementum in older individuals is the usual and expected condition. Such cementum exposure is frequently seen to a some degree on the maxillary canines or other teeth of persons younger than 30 years of age. After the age of 30, cementum exposure increases in frequency and extent. By 40 years of age, cementum is exposed on some areas of most of the teeth of many individuals. By age 60, cementum exposure in some areas may extend 3 or 4 mm (Fig. 11-3). An individual of middle age with no cementum exposed on any teeth is unusual.

CLINICAL CONSIDERATIONS

The intactness of the epithelium of the gingival sulcus and junctional epithelium is important to good periodontal health. Because the gingival sulcus, despite the snug fit of the free gingiva to the tooth surface, is exposed to the saliva and microorganisms of the oral cavity, damage to the epithelium of the gingival sulcus can result in damage to the underlying connective tissue. Unlike epithelium, connective tissue is not a covering tissue and does not resist injury and microorganism invasion. Therefore, if damage to the epithelium of the gingival sulcus is accompanied by damage to the underlying connective tissue, the ensuing effect on the tissues in this area may include inflammation, swelling, damage to the periodontal ligament fibers, resorption of the bone of the alveolar process, and loosening of the tooth. As a result, tooth removal may be necessary.

The presence of calculus around the cervix of a tooth is often an important factor in periodontal disease. Calculus damages the epithelium of the gingival sulcus and junctional epithelium and results in the following series of events: inflammation of the connective tissue of the gingiva; swelling; damage to the periodontal ligament fibers, particularly the gingival, transseptal, and alveolar crest fibers; resorption of the bone of the alveolar crest; and an increasing amount of exposed cementum in the cervical area of the tooth.

Figure 11-14 is a drawing of the cervical area on the lingual side of a maxillary molar. The periodontium is in good condition, and little or no inflammation is seen in the gingiva. The junctional epithelium fits against the tooth; the periodontal ligament fibers are well oriented; and the alveolar crest shows no signs of resorption.

Figure 11-15 is a drawing of the cervical area on the buccal side of the same tooth. The presence of a mass of calculus has caused a gingival pocket to form. The result has been injury to the epithelium of the gingival sulcus, inflammation in the connective tissue, damage to the periodontal ligament fibers, and resorption of the alveolar crest and lamina dura. Continued irritation by the calculus will be accompanied by continued inflammation of the gingiva and continued bone resorption. Such pathosis, when sufficiently extended, results in the loosening of the tooth.

Figure 11-16 is a photomicrograph of a section of the lingual side of a maxillary molar and associated periodontium. No calculus is observed on the tooth surface, and little inflammation is observed in the gingiva. Compare this tooth with the one in Figures 11-14 and 11-15.

Another important clinical problem is created by the presence in the mouth of exposed cervical cementum. When the exposed cervical cementum extends beyond 1 mm, a condition known as *cervical abrasion* frequently is found. Cervical abrasion is a wedge-shaped cut in the cervical cementum of a tooth that is produced when the person uses an abrasive dentifrice and brushes the teeth with a cross-brushing stroke. Although the tooth enamel, because of its extreme hardness, is not affected by this procedure, the cementum is abraded. Cervical abrasion is seen in its most severe form in mouths that are consistently kept clean and on the facial sides of the teeth, where the most vigorous brushing occurs. A study of cervical abrasion demonstrated that in 7.6 years use of a cross-brushing technique with an abrasive dentifrice can cause a maxillary canine tooth measuring 7 mm at the cervix to be cut halfway through. During that time, the wedge of cervical abrasion can extend halfway through the 7-mm cervix. Figure 11-3 is a clinical photo-

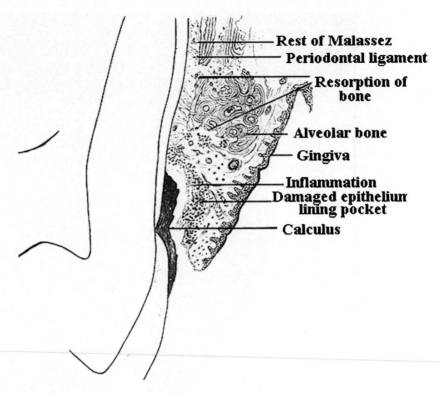

Figure 11–15. Diagrammatic drawing of the facial side of the tooth illustrated in Fig. 11-14. A large mass of calculus at the tooth cervix is responsible for the pathologic condition in this area. Inflammation, destruction of the junctional epithelium, damage to the periodontal ligament, and resorption of the alveolar crest and lamina dura are observed.

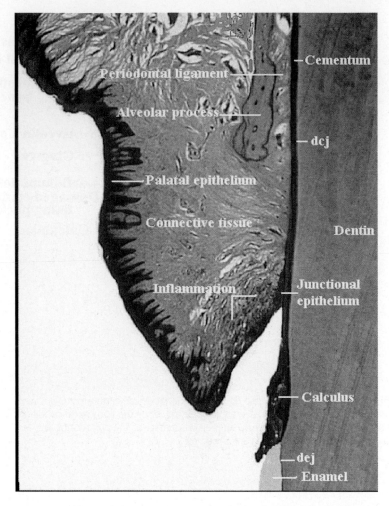

Figure 11–16. Faciolingual histologic section of gingiva and adjacent tissue. This figure reveals a condition frequently encountered in clinical practice—calculus-causing gingival inflammation.

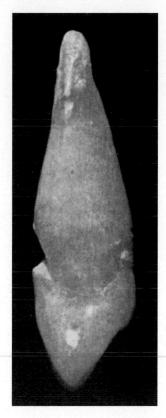

Figure 11–17. Mesial surface of a maxillary canine tooth. Deep abrasion of the cervical cementum is observed on the facial surface. The enamel is not affected. Sclerotic and reparative dentin (see Fig. 5-22) ordinarily form beneath such an area of abrasion.

graph that shows cervical abrasion. Figure 11-17 depicts an extracted maxillary canine tooth with deep cervical abrasion. Figure 5-22 also shows a ground section of a mandibular incisor tooth in which slight cervical abrasion is observed on the labial side, with dead tract and sclerotic dentin beneath.

Such information concerning cervical abrasion makes clear the importance of using proper toothbrushing techniques and a dentifrice that does not contain an excessive amount of abrasive material. This information is particularly important for individuals in whom considerable gingival recession has exposed a relatively broad area of cementum to the oral cavity.

SUGGESTED READINGS

Carranza FA Jr, ed. Glickman's Clinical Periodontology. 7th ed. Philadelphia (PA): WB Saunders; 1990.
Schroeder HE, Listgarten MA. The gingival tissues: the architecture of periodontal protection. Periodontol 2000 1997;13:91–120.

12 *The Salivary Glands*

Salivary glands are exocrine glands that secrete a colorless, slightly sticky fluid called saliva into the oral cavity through ducts that open onto the surface of the oral mucosa. Saliva is a critical component of oral and dental health. Disruption in salivary flow due to disease, drugs, or radiation therapy not only can have dire effects on the teeth and oral mucosa, but it also can reduce patients' overall quality of life by reducing their ability to eat and speak. Disruption of salivary gland function can upset the ecological balance of microorganisms in the oral cavity and lead to a dramatic increase in caries, periodontal disease, and oral yeast (*Candida albicans*) infections.

DEVELOPMENT OF SALIVARY GLANDS

Salivary glands, like teeth (See Chapter 3), originate from interactions between the oral ectoderm and branchial arch mesenchyme. The ectodermal cells give rise to the parenchyma of the gland that ultimately forms both the secretory and ductal cells (Fig. 12-1). Meanwhile, the mesenchyme forms the connective tissue stroma that supports the gland and provides access for the vasculature and nerves that supply it.

Initiation of salivary gland development begins when the oral ectoderm grows into the underlying connective tissue during the sixth to twelfth weeks of embryonic development. Six buds are formed at specified sites and ultimately mark the exit point of each main excretory duct for the paired parotid, submandibular (submaxillary), and sublingual glands (Fig. 12-2). Additional buds scattered on the tongue, lips, buccal mucosa, and palate give rise to *minor salivary glands* distributed beneath the oral mucous membranes. As the epithelial cells grow into the connective tissue and multiply, they form both the secretory cells that produce saliva and the system of ductal cells that transmit and modify the saliva before it reaches the oral cavity.

DISTRIBUTION OF SALIVARY GLANDS

Major salivary glands are paired organs (Fig. 12-2). The largest glands are the *parotid glands* located under the skin of the face, in front of the ear, and above the angle of the jaw. Human parotid glands produce watery or serous saliva. The main duct of each parotid gland, the *parotid duct (Stensen's duct)*, opens into the oral cavity on the wall of either cheek opposite the maxillary second molar tooth. If the

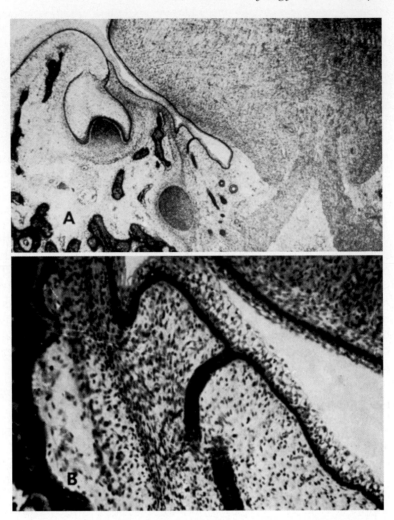

Figure 12–1. Photomicrograph of a frontal section of one side of the lower jaw of a 5-month-old human fetus. **A.** The tongue (right) and the tooth germ of a posterior tooth (left) can clearly seen. From the oral epithelium under the tongue, a slender growth of epithelial cells curves downward into the connective tissue. This is the beginning of the development of a salivary gland and its secretory duct. The two small circles beneath the tongue are cross sections of two salivary gland ducts, which are parts of the larger Wharton's duct. **B.** A higher magnification of the area under the tongue.

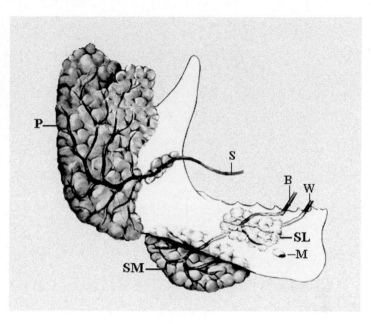

Figure 12–2. Anatomical position of the three major salivary glands in relation to a lateral view of the mandible. P, parotid gland; S, Stensen's duct; SM, submandibular gland; W, Wharton's duct; SL, sublingual gland; B, Batholin's duct; and M, mental foramen.

tongue is passed over this area, a small prominence may be felt where the duct opens into the mouth. The parotid gland is involved in epidemic parotitis, commonly known as mumps.

Submandibular glands are located beneath the floor of the mouth in depressions on the lingual surfaces of the mandible, just anterior to the angle of the jaw. This gland produces a mixture of serous and mucous saliva that gains entry to the oral cavity through the submandibular ducts (*Wharton's ducts*). These ducts open into the floor of the mouth beneath the tongue, one on either side of the midline. These duct openings are clearly seen as two small prominences in this area.

Sublingual glands are the smallest of the major salivary glands. They are located above the floor of the mouth, beneath the mucosa that lines the floor of the mouth, but anterior to the submandibular glands. These glands produce a mixture of mucous and serous saliva. In contrast to the other major glands, sublingual secretions are delivered to the mouth through several main ducts. Some of these ducts open along the crest of the plica sublingualis, whereas others join the submandibular ducts and share the same openings. Examine carefully the area under the tongue in a human mouth.

Minor salivary glands are generally described according to their location in the oral cavity. Beneath the mucous membrane of the cheeks and lips are numerous small glands composed of both mucous and serous secretory cells; the mucous cells are the more numerous (Fig. 12-3). The minute duct openings of these small glands are scattered over the surface of the cheek and lip mucosa. Larger salivary glands composed entirely of mucous cells lie beneath the mucous membrane of the roof of the mouth and have minute duct openings that are distributed over the entire surface of the hard and soft palate. The tongue contains glands in its anterior part that also contain both serous and mucous cells. In the posterior part of the

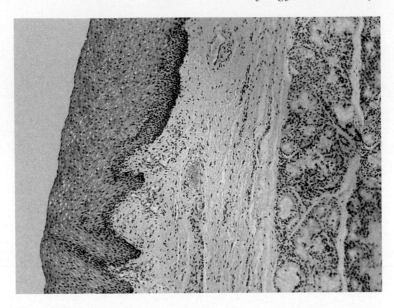

Figure 12–3. Histologic section of the buccal mucosa of the cheek. Interposed between a minor salivary gland (right) and the darkly stained oral mucosa (left) is the lighter stained lamina propria or connective tissue.

tongue, *von Ebner's glands* are composed entirely of serous cells; ducts of these glands empty into the trenches of the circumvallate papillae. Glands composed purely of mucous cells also are found in the root of the tongue and in the floor of the mouth (Table 12-1).

In the cheeks and lips, a thick submucosa contains fat tissue and many salivary glands with minute duct openings that are scattered over the surface of the mucosa. Occasionally, what appears to be a pea-sized bubble just beneath the surface of the mucosa can be seen. When one of these small salivary ducts becomes blocked, the secretion from a salivary gland accumulates near the surface. This bubble is called a *mucocele*.[1]

HISTOLOGY OF SALIVARY GLANDS

Each salivary gland is composed of a complex array of ducts that terminate as blind pouches surrounded by a small cluster of secretory cells. A single cluster is referred to as an *acinus* because of its grape-like appearance. These acini are composed of serous cells, mucous cells, or a combination of both. In the parotid gland, the acini are composed solely of serous cells (Fig. 12-4). The submandibular glands also predominantly contain serous acini but are interspersed with clusters of mucous-producing cells (Figs. 12-5 and 12-6). In contrast, although it contains a few serous cells, the sublingual gland is primarily composed of mucous acini (Fig. 12-7 and 12-8).

The lumen of each acinus is continuous with a duct system. This system exhibits unique architectural features along its length, and in it three levels of or-

---

[1] Pronounced *mū′ kō sĕl.*

TABLE 12–1. Classification of Salivary Glands

Glands	Secretory Cells	Secretions	Main Ducts	Mucosa Sites of Duct Openings
Major:				
parotid	serous	serous	Stensen's	lining
submandibular	serous mucous	seromucous	Wharton's	lining
sublingual	serous mucous	seromucous	Bartholin's	lining
Minor:				
lips and cheeks	serous mucous	seromucous		lining
sublingual	mucous	mucous		lining
glossopharyngeal	mucous	mucous		lining
hard palate	mucous	mucous		masticatory
soft palate	mucous	mucous		lining
anterior tongue	serous mucous	seromucous		lining
middle tongue	serous	serous		specialized
posterior tongue	mucous	mucous		specialized

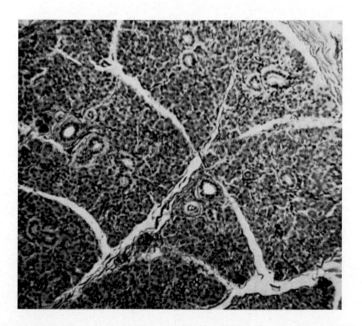

Figure 12–4. Photomicrograph of a human parotid gland (low power). The secretory cells are all serous. In several places, cross sections of the ducts of this gland are seen. They appear in this view as circular openings lined with cuboidal epithelial cells. These small ducts coalesce into larger ducts, which empty the gland secretions into the mouth at openings located on the inside of the cheek.

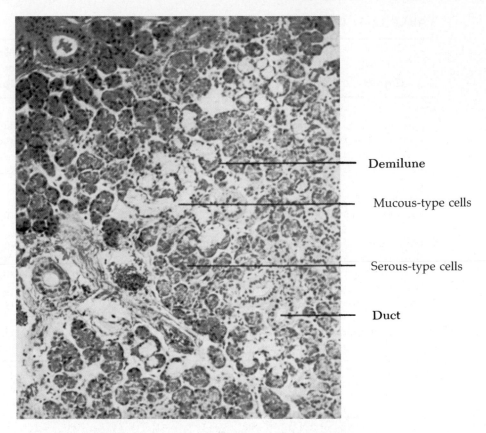

Figure 12–5. Photomicrograph of a histologic section of a human submandibular gland. Both serous and mucous secretory cells are present; the serous type is more numerous. The groups of light-colored mucous cells (center) in some cases are capped on one side by serous cells. In histologic sections, these capping cells have the shape of a "new moon," and some imaginative histologists have called them demilunes (demi = half; lunes = moons). Cross sections of ducts are seen in the section.

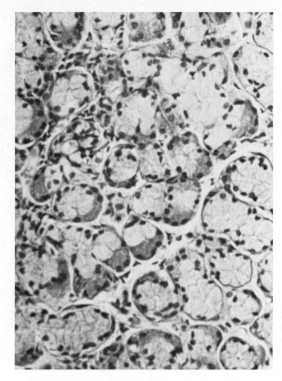

Figure 12–6. Higher magnification of a section of a human submandibular gland. The darker cells are the serous cells of demilunes; the lighter-stained cells are mucous cells.

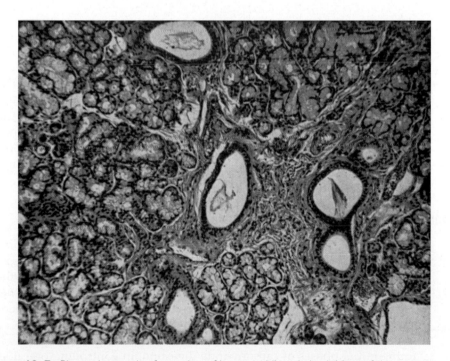

Figure 12–7. Photomicrograph of a section of human sublingual gland. Most of the secretory cells here are of mucous cells; the darker-stained serous cells are sparingly scattered in the gland, often in the form of demilunes. Cross sections of ducts are also seen in this figure. The large openings represent excretory ducts.

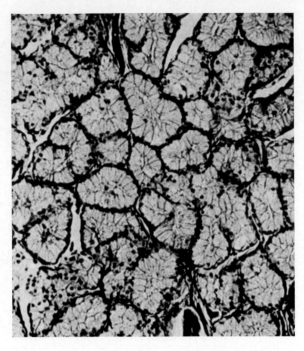

Figure 12–8. Photomicrograph of a section of a minor sublingual gland from the floor of the mouth. All the secretory cells here are of the mucous type.

ganization can be histologically identified. The transition from the lumen to the *intercalated duct* is marked by a change from the secretory cells of the acinus to low cuboidal cells that contain centrally located nuclei (Fig. 12-9). Continuing towards the mouth, the next duct is the *striated duct* (Fig.12-9). Striated ducts are lined by columnar epithelium cells with apically positioned nuclei and a striated border along the basal end of the cell. *Excretory ducts* comprise the transition between the striated ducts and the stratified epithelium of the oral cavity (Fig. 12-7). Remote from the mouth, the excretory ducts are lined by a pseudostratified columnar epithelium, whereas near the orifice of the duct they are lined by a true stratified epithelium.

COMPOSITION AND FUNCTION OF SALIVA

The total volume of saliva produced by the salivary glands varies from individual to individual, but averages approximately is 1 liter per day. Saliva is a mixture of water, ions, and various proteins produced by the secretory cells in the acini and modified by the ductal cells en route to the oral cavity. Saliva is further modified when it reaches the mouth by the addition of crevicular fluid, oral microbes, white blood cells, and desquamated epithelial cells.

Saliva has multiple functions in the oral cavity. Salivary proteins are important in the initial phases of carbohydrate digestion, in controlling oral microbes, and maintaining the structural integrity of the tooth surface by enhancing remineralization. In addition, the water phase of saliva lubricates oral tissue (thus assisting

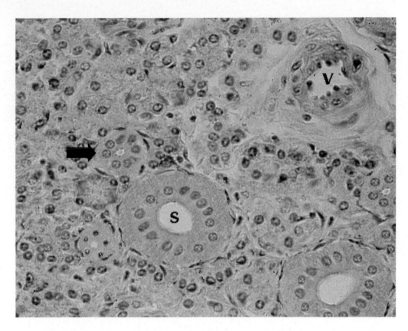

Figure 12–9. (See Color Plates) High magnification of salivary gland ducts. The arrow points to an intercalated duct. A striated duct lumen (S) and the lumen of a blood vessel (V) are labeled for comparison.

in mastication and speech), serves as a solvent for tastants, and helps to flush debris from the oral cavity.

SUGGESTED READINGS

Atkinson JC, Wu AJ. Salivary gland dysfunction: causes, symptoms, treatment. J Am Dent Assoc 1994;125:409–416.

Fox PC. Management of dry mouth. Dent Clin North Am 1997;41:863–875.

Grisius MM, Fox PC. Salivary gland dysfunction and xerostomia. In: Linden RW, ed. Frontiers in Oral Biology. New York (NY): Basel Karger; 1998: 156–167.

13 Tooth Eruption and the Shedding of the Primary Teeth

TOOTH ERUPTION

Tooth eruption is the combination of bodily movements of the tooth, both before and after the tooth crown emerges into the oral cavity. It serves to bring and maintain the tooth in occlusion with the teeth of the opposing arch. Tooth eruption begins when crown formation is completed and the root begins to form and continues throughout the life of the tooth.

ERUPTIVE MOVEMENTS

In its simplest form, tooth eruption may be pictured as the occlusal movement of the tooth. Such movement results, at least in part, from the lengthening of the root and the development of additional bone beneath the root. During the process of root eruption, the root does not grow deeper into the jaw; instead, the position of the apical end of the developing root remains relatively fixed. As the developing root lengthens, its growing apical end maintains its position, and the crown moves occlusally. This description provides an oversimplified picture of the process, however, because teeth without roots can erupt and because teeth can erupt over a distance greater than the length of their roots.

During the development of the permanent dentition, the movements of tooth eruption vary. Movement may be relatively slight, such as in the relatively simple process of occlusal movement in the anterior teeth. Movement may also occur through a condition of considerable horizontal movement, such as in the premolars, or through a highly complex set of rotating and horizontal movements, such as in the molars.

With the exception of the enamel of permanent molar teeth, the enamel organ of each permanent tooth develops from the dental lamina lingual to its primary predecessor (see Figs. 3-15, 3-16, and 3-17). By the time the primary tooth has emerged into the oral cavity, the development of the permanent tooth is well advanced. In the anterior region, the permanent teeth continue development lingual to their primary predecessors. However, in the region of the premolars, a change in relative position occurs: the premolars replace the primary molars. By the time the primary molars have come into occlusion, the crowns of the developing premolars occupy a position not lingual to, but between the roots of, the primary molars (Figs. 13-1, 13-2, 13-3, and 13-4). This change in relative positions occurs as a

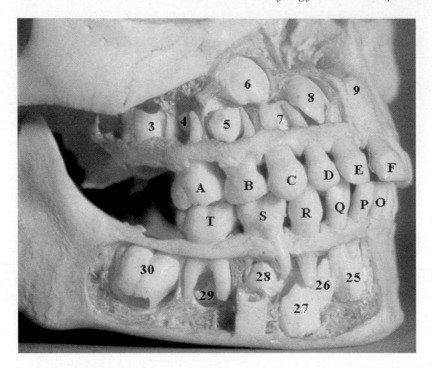

Figure 13–1. Lateral view of a 4-year-old skull with the facial aspect of the maxillary and mandibular alveolar processes removed. Notice that the primary teeth have erupted and are in occlusion and that their roots are intact. Observe the positions of the succedaneous tooth crowns and their relationship to the primary tooth roots. The positions of the permanent canines (6 and 27) are conspicuous. Crowns of the first permanent molars (3 and 30) lie distal to the roots of the primary second molars (A and T). The permanent molars, including the second and third molars which are not present here, are not succedaneous teeth. Compare this skull to the 5-year-old skull in Figs. 13-2 and 13-3.

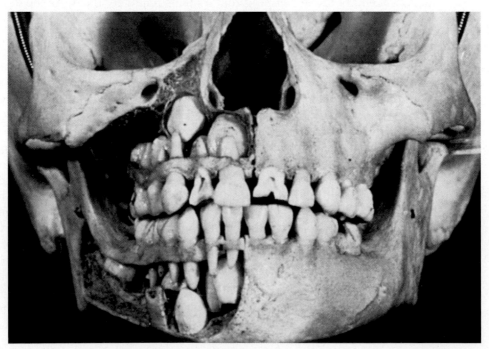

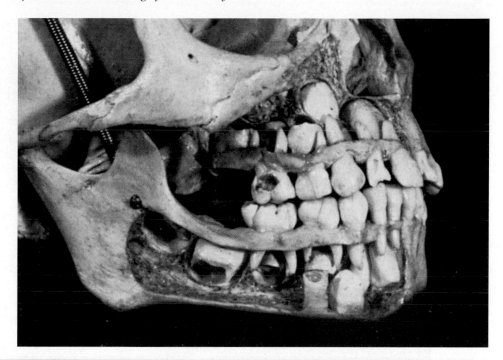

Figure 13–3. Lateral view of the posterior region of the skull seen in Fig. 13-2. Crowns of the premolars are seen between the roots of the primary molars. Note the buccal caries in the primary maxillary second molar. Crowns of the permanent first molars are surrounded by bone and located distal to the roots of the primary second molars. The developing crown of the mandibular permanent second molar is seen in its bone crypt, just distal to the permanent first molar crown. Compare to Figs. 13-1 and 13-4.

Figure 13–2. Anterior view of a 5-year-old dry skull. The right facial cortical plate of the maxillary and mandibular bones has been removed to show the developing permanent teeth and their relationship to the primary teeth. Crowns of the permanent anterior teeth are located lingual to the roots of the primary anterior teeth. Note the relation of the permanent maxillary central incisor to the floor of the nasal cavity; also note the permanent maxillary canine crown and its relation to the orbit of the eye. The permanent mandibular anterior teeth bear a close relationship to one another. Note the lingual position of the mandibular permanent lateral incisor. Compare to Figs. 13-1 and 13-4.

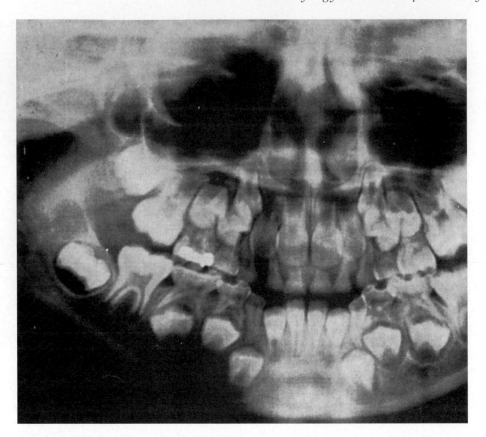

Figure 13–4. Panoramic radiograph of a child at approximately 6 years of age. The permanent mandibular incisors and the permanent maxillary and mandibular first molars are present in the oral cavity. The permanent maxillary central incisors, with roots still short and root canals broad, lie above the partially resorbed roots of the primary incisors. Primary teeth still present in the oral cavity are maxillary incisors, canines, and first and second molars; those in the lower jaw are canines and first and second molars. Crowns of the permanent canines and first and second molars and their relationship to the primary teeth they will replace are best seen in the lower jaw (left).

Crowns of the developing maxillary and mandibular permanent second molars lie in a bone crypt distal to the erupted first molars; roots have not begun to form. Distal to the crown of the permanent mandibular second molar (left) is a light circle of bone enclosing a dark area, which is the location of the forming third molar.

Above the forming roots of the permanent maxillary incisors is the nasal cavity; on either side of the nasal cavity are the orbits of the eye (large dark areas). The forming roots of the right and left permanent maxillary canines have an interesting and important relationship to the nasal cavity and eye orbits. (Courtesy Dr. Gus Pappas, College of Dentistry, Ohio State University.)

result of a vertical movement of the primary teeth and a horizontal movement of the developing permanent teeth. The portion of the permanent dentition that replaces the primary dentition is referred to as the *succedaneous dentition*.

Permanent molar teeth do not have predecessors, and the enamel organs of permanent molar tooth germs develop from an extension of the dental lamina distal to the position of the primary molars. The first permanent molars develop in approximately the position they will hold upon emergence into the oral cavity. However, the crowns of the second and third molars form in a different position and must undergo complicated motions of rotation and forward movement to emerge into correct relation to other teeth.

When the second and third molars begin to develop, neither the maxilla nor the mandible is large enough to accommodate them. Therefore , the mandibular second and third molars develop in the ramus of the mandible, with their occlusal surfaces directed mesially. The second molar usually emerges into the oral cavity in its correct position distal to the first molar. However, inadequate jaw development and a failure of sufficient rotating movement in the early stages of eruption sometimes cause the crown of the mandibular third molar to press against the roots of the adjacent second molar. The result of such a positional relationship is an impacted third molar. Figure 13-5 shows a mandibular third molar crown forming in the usual position in the *ramus of the mandible*.

In the maxilla, the second and third molars develop in the *maxillary tuberosity*, with their occlusal surfaces directed distally and buccally. Inadequate jaw development and a failure of sufficient rotating movement in the early stages of eruption may result in the emergence of the maxillary third molar with its occlusal surface directed distally and buccally. The change in position of developing teeth in the jaws is a result of the growth of the teeth, alveolar process, and jaws (Fig. 13-5). Figure 13-6 is a histologic section through the region of a mandibular third molar that is in a position similar to the position of the lower third molar seen in Figure 13-5.

During tooth eruption, the tooth emerges into the oral cavity. Figure 13-7 is a diagram of several events involved in this emergence. In Figure 13-7A, the tooth crown is complete, but root formation has not yet begun. The reduced enamel epithelium covering the crown is separated from the epithelium that lines the oral cavity by an area of connective tissue. In Figure 13-7B, root formation is in

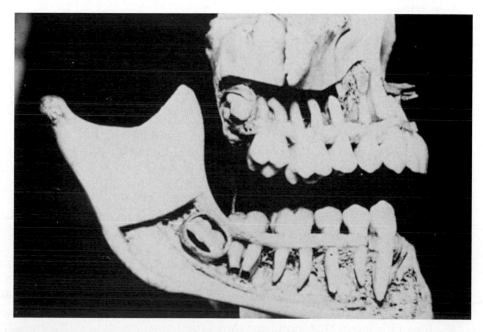

Figure 13–5. A human maxilla and mandible with the facial parts of the alveolar process removed, except near the cervical border. Notice the location and position of the developing mandibular and maxillary third molars. The crown of the mandibular third molar is nearly complete in the ramus of the mandible. Its occlusal surface is directed mesially and occlusally, and it is surrounded by a bone crypt. The maxillary third molar is directed buccally and distally.

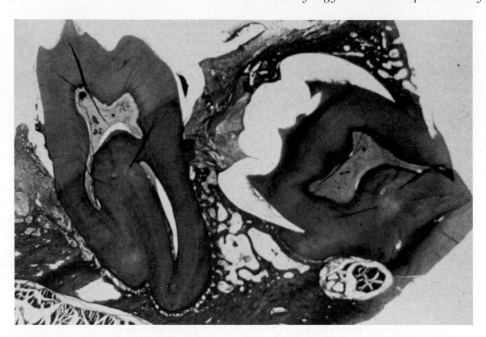

Figure 13–6. Histologic section of a lower third molar region. The third molar, the occlusal surface of which is directed mesially, is surrounded by bone of the mandible. Note the third molar's relation to the erupted second molar. The enamel of the two teeth was completely demineralized during processing. Interestingly, the enamel "space" (white area) of the third molar retains the original enamel outline because of the surrounding bone. Compare to Fig. 13-5.

progress, and the crown has moved occlusally. Following the occlusal movement of the tooth crown, the reduced enamel epithelium has come into contact with the oral epithelium. At the cervical border of the reduced enamel epithelium, some cells appear to have broken off and remain an open network of epithelial cells in the periodontal ligament surrounding the tooth root. This network is *Hertwig's epithelial sheath*. In Figure 13-7C, the epithelial cells that previously covered the incisal edge of the tooth have been penetrated, and the tip of the tooth has become visible in the mouth. After the tooth emerges into the mouth, the reduced enamel epithelium becomes known as the *junctional epithelium* (see Fig. 13-7D), but this change is merely one of terminology. With age, the cells at the apical end of the junctional epithelium proliferate onto the cementum of the root (see Figs. 13-7E and 11-12).

Figure 13-8 is a diagrammatic illustration of the process of root formation and eruption of a two-rooted tooth. The process is similar to that for a single-rooted tooth illustrated in Figure 13-7.

Although the tooth comes into occlusion during root formation, occlusal movement does not cease when the root is completed. Because of changes in the surrounding bone, and perhaps also because of continued cementum formation at the root end, occlusal movement may continue, at least intermittently, throughout the life of the tooth. This continued slow eruption serves an important need. Because years of use may cause the occlusal and incisal areas of the teeth to be considerably worn off, continued occlusal movement of the teeth during advancing years helps to compensate for loss of crown length.

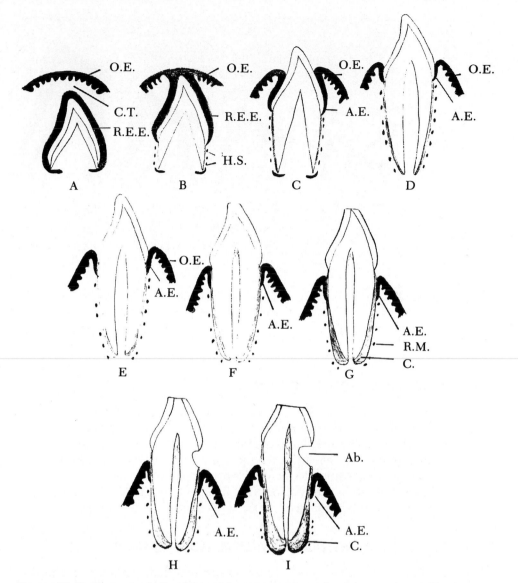

Figure 13–7. Diagrammatic illustration of the process of root formation, tooth eruption, the rootward migration of the attachment epithelium, cementum exposure, and cervical abrasion. **A.** The reduced enamel epithelium covers the tooth crown and is separated from the oral epithelium by connective tissue. The root has not yet begun to form. **B.** Root formation has begun, and the crown has moved incisally. The reduced enamel and oral epithelia are in contact. **C.** The root is longer, and the incisal edge of the crown is exposed in the oral cavity. The reduced enamel epithelium, which is the remains of the enamel organ, is now continuous with the oral epithelium and is called the junctional epithelium. **D.** The length of the root dentin is complete, and the crown has moved farther into the oral cavity. The junctional epithelium is still entirely on the enamel. The apical foramen is narrower. **E–G.** The junctional epithelium grows onto the cementum at its apical border and separates from the tooth surface at its cervical border. Cementum becomes exposed. **H, I.** Increased cementum exposure and improper use of an abrasive dentifrice have resulted in abrasion of cementum and dentin in the cervical area. OE, oral epithelium; CT, connective tissue; REE, reduced enamel epithelium; HS, Hertwig's sheath; AE, attachment (junctional) epithelium; RM, rests of Malassez; C, cementum; and AB, abrasion.

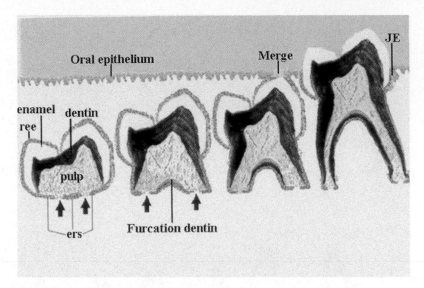

Figure 13–8. Diagrammatic illustration of the process of root formation and eruption of a two-rooted tooth. The descriptions for a single-rooted tooth which illustrated in Fig. 13-7A–13-7D can also be cited for this figure. The arrows indicate the openings in the epithelial root sheath that indicate the future formation of root canals. REE, reduced enamel epithelium; ERS, epithelial (Hertwig's) root sheath.

THE MECHANISM OF TOOTH ERUPTION

The mechanism of tooth eruption is difficult to explain. Early occlusal movement appears to result from a combination of factors. First, the tissue beneath the growing root resists the apical movement of the developing root. This resistance results in the occlusal movement of the tooth crown as the root lengthens. Second, bone formation occurs apical to the developing tooth. Other factors involved are vascular pressures within the periodontal ligament and traction by the cells and fibers of the periodontal ligament.

CERVICAL EXPOSURE WITHOUT OCCLUSAL MOVEMENT

In young individuals, tooth crowns are smaller than anatomic crowns (Fig. 13-7C). As people age, the length of the clinical crown usually increases because some cervical cementum is exposed to the oral cavity (see Fig. 11-3), and more cementum exposure occurs through the years than can be accounted for by actual occlusal tooth movement. Although the teeth undoubtedly undergo occlusal movement, part of their increased exposure throughout life results from progressive loss of soft tissue attachment. This loss occurs when the apical end of the junctional (attachment) epithelium, which originally was located at the cementoenamel junction, proliferates or grows onto the cementum (see Figs. 13-7E and 11-14). In addition, the coronal end of the attachment, which is the bottom of the gingival sulcus, likewise moves apically. To a limited degree, the apical migration of the junctional epithelium is a normal condition. This apical movement of the gingiva is called *gingival recession.*

Eventually, cementum is exposed at the cervix of the tooth (see Fig. 13-7G). Exposed cementum is found both in the mouths of nearly all individuals older than 40 years of age and in the mouths of many younger individuals.

MESIAL DRIFT

Several tooth movements have already been mentioned: the easily recognized occlusal movement of the erupting tooth; the horizontal movements that place the developing crowns of permanent premolars between the roots of the primary molars; and the complicated combination of rotating and lateral movements that brings second and third molars into their functional position.

In addition to these tooth movements, another type of tooth movement known as *mesial drift* occurs. Mesial drift is the lateral bodily movement of teeth on both sides of the mouth toward the midline of the arch. One condition that leads to mesial drift may be understood by picturing the teeth in function. Because teeth are suspended in their sockets by the fibers of the periodontal ligament, they are not rigid in the jaws but undergo considerable movement during mastication. This functional movement produces a rubbing of the contact areas. Some evidence shows that, as the proximal surfaces of adjacent teeth become worn from functional tooth movement, the transseptal fibers of the periodontal ligament become shorter and thereby maintain tooth contact.

Mesial drift is possible because of the adaptability of bone tissue. Pressure on the periodontal ligament fibers results in resorption of bone, whereas pull on fibers results in bone apposition (formation). As the contact areas of the crowns wear, the teeth tend to move mesially, thereby maintaining contact. The slight pressure thus produced on the mesial side of the socket results in slow resorption of the lamina dura. The accompanying tension of the periodontal ligament fibers on the distal side of the root induces appositional lamina dura bone in this area. As a consequence of these bone changes, an actual shift in the position of the tooth socket occurs.

SHEDDING OF THE PRIMARY TEETH

Primary and Permanent Dentitions

The human *primary dentition* is made of one central incisor, one lateral incisor, one canine, and two molar teeth in each quadrant of the mouth. The first teeth to become visible in the oral cavity usually are the primary mandibular central incisors, which emerge when the child is approximately 6 months old. The last primary teeth to appear are the maxillary second molars, which appear at approximately the end of the second year. Each tooth of the primary dentition is eventually lost and replaced by a tooth of the permanent dentition.

The *permanent dentition* consists of one central incisor, one lateral incisor, one canine, two premolars, and three molars in each quadrant of the mouth. The first permanent tooth to appear usually is a first molar, which emerges just behind the second primary molar when the child is approximately 6 years of age. The last primary tooth to remain in the mouth usually is the second primary molar, which is replaced by the permanent second premolar in approximately the twelfth year. The permanent molars have no predecessors. The first permanent molars appear in the mouth during the sixth year, when the primary dentition may still be intact, but they must be recognized as teeth of the permanent dentition and not regarded as primary teeth soon to be lost.

Table 13-1 lists the times of emergence into the oral cavity of the teeth of the primary and permanent dentitions, as well as the times of the beginning of hard tissue formation in each of the teeth.

TABLE 13–1. The Chronology of the Human Dentition

		Tooth	Formation of Enamel Matrix and Dentin Begins	Time of Emergence Into Oral Cavity
Primary dentition	Maxillary	Central incisor	4 mos. in utero	7½ mos.
		Lateral incisor	4½ mos. in utero	9 mos.
		Canine	5 mos. in utero	18 mos.
		First molar	5 mos. in utero	14 mos.
		Second molar	6 mos. in utero	24 mos.
	Mandibular	Central incisor	4½ mos. in utero	6 mos.
		Lateral incisor	4½ mos. in utero	7 mos.
		Canine	5 mos. in utero	16 mos.
		First molar	5 mos. in utero	12 mos.
		Second molar	6 mos. in utero	20 mos.
Permanent dentition	Maxillary	Central incisor	3–4 mos.	7–8 yrs.
		Lateral incisor	10–12 mos.	8–9 yrs.
		Canine	4–5 mos.	11–12 yrs.
		First premolar	1½–1¾ yrs.	10–11 yrs.
		Second premolar	2–2¼ yrs.	10–12 yrs.
		First molar	At birth	6–7 yrs.
		Second molar	2½–3 yrs.	12–13 yrs.
		Third molar	7–9 yrs.	17–21 yrs.
	Mandibular	Central incisor	3–4 mos.	6–7 yrs.
		Lateral incisor	3–4 mos.	7–8 yrs.
		Canine	4–5 mos.	9–10 yrs.
		First premolar	1¾–2 yrs.	10–12 yrs.
		Second premolar	2¼–2½ yrs.	11–12 yrs.
		First molar	At birth	6–7 yrs.
		Second molar	2½–3 yrs.	11–13 yrs.
		Third molar	8–10 yrs.	17–21 yrs.

Adapted from Orban after Logan and Kronfeld (slightly modified by McCall and Schour).

THE PROCESS OF SHEDDING

The shedding of primary teeth is the result of the gradual *resorption* of their roots and the consequent loss of periodontal ligament attachment. The increase in size of the developing permanent successor, which is located lingual to (beneath) the root of the functioning primary tooth, most likely creates sufficient pressure to produce resorption of the primary tooth root and surrounding bone (Figs. 13-9, 13-10, and 13-11). As the root resorbs, the tooth loosens. Eventually, all periodontal ligament attachment is lost, and the rootless crown of the primary tooth literally falls off the jaw.

Figure 13–10. Radiograph of the lower anterior region of the mouth. The positions of the permanent incisors apical to the resorbed roots of the shedding primary incisors are illustrated.

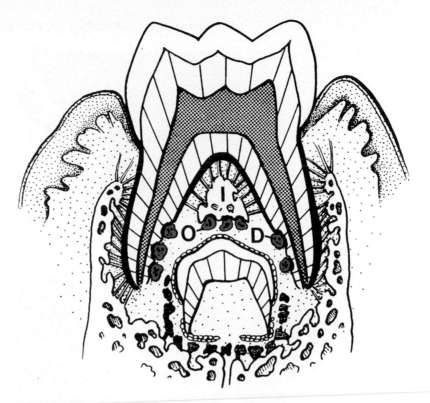

Figure 13–9. Diagram of the early shedding stage of a primary tooth and the position of a permanent tooth between its roots. Dentinoclasts (D) are seen along the interradicular surfaces of the apical root area; osteoclasts (O) are present along the interradicular bone (I) of the primary tooth. Notice the arrangement of the clast cells along the surface toward which the permanent tooth is erupting.

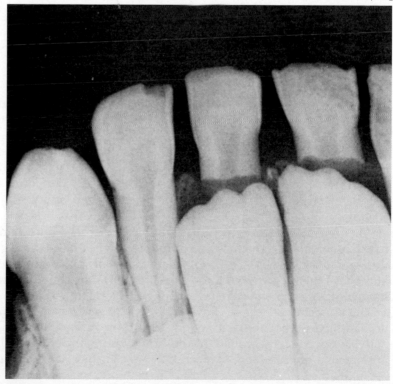

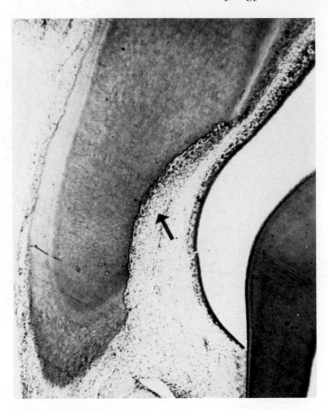

Figure 13–11. Section of the apical end of a primary tooth and its succedaneous (permanent) tooth located between the primary tooth roots. A concave resorption area is clearly seen on the primary root (arrow), just adjacent to the permanent tooth crown (right). Resorption has advanced to the root dentin, and the cementum of the area has been resorbed. Notice the reduced enamel epithelium over the enamel of the permanent tooth. See Fig. 13-9 for a gross view of shedding.

The mineralized tissues of primary tooth roots, cementum, and dentin are physiologically resorbed by large, multinucleated cells (Figs. 13-12 and 13-13). These cells resemble an osteoclast (see Fig. 9-14), which is the cell responsible for bone resorption. The cell that resorbs the mineralized tissues of a tooth is called an *odontoclast*. When the odontoclast resorbs cementum, it may be called a *cementoclast*; when it resorbs dentin, it may be called a *dentinoclast*. In Figure 13-14, cementoclasts and dentinoclasts are found along the root of a primary tooth undergoing shedding.

An interesting phenomenon that is frequently observed in children is the alternate loosening and tightening of a primary tooth before it is finally shed. One day, the child reports a loose tooth, but several days later the tooth appears to be firmly attached. When resorption of the primary tooth root causes the tooth to become loose, not only is pressure relieved, but slight tension also appears to be induced on the adjacent connective tissue. This tension stimulates the connective tissue around the resorbed root end to form new cementum on the remaining root end and new bone to form around the root. Therefore, new periodontal ligament fibers are attached, and the tooth tightens in the jaw. Further development of the perma-

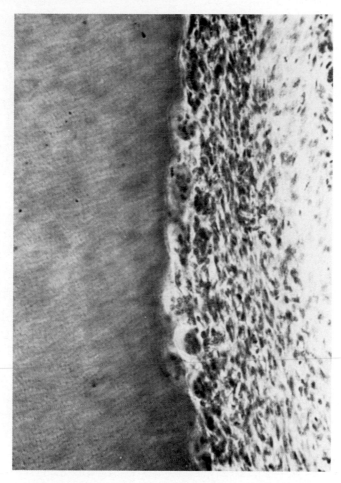

Figure 13–12. Higher magnification of the concave resorption area of the primary tooth root seen in Fig. 13-11. Dentinoclasts lie along the surface of the root dentin.

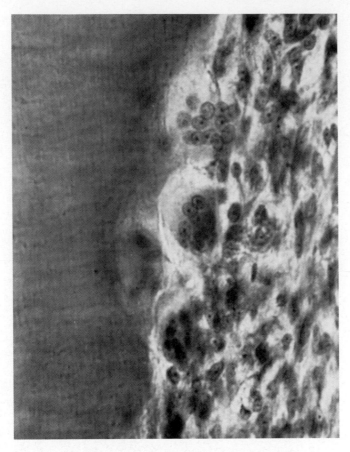

Figure 13–13. Higher magnification of the resorption area seen in Fig. 13-12. Three multinucleated dentinoclasts are clearly visible. Note how these cells fit into the cupped-out sites of the dentin at which resorption is occurring.

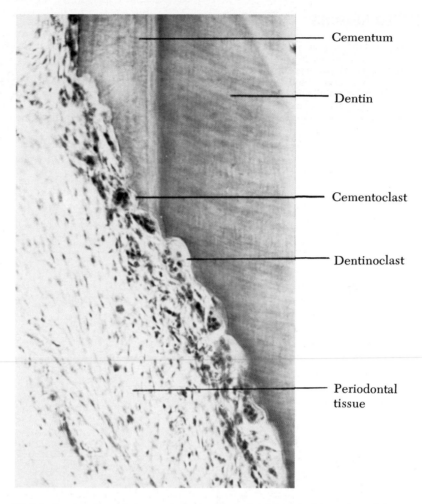

Cementum

Dentin

Cementoclast

Dentinoclast

Periodontal
tissue

Figure 13–14. Section through the root of a shedding primary tooth. Resorption of cementum and dentin is well advanced. Cementoclasts and dentinoclasts are found within resorption sites along the root. Where would the permanent tooth be located?

nent tooth soon causes more resorption of both bone and root. Although loosening and reattachment may alternate several times, as the permanent tooth continues to develop, the accompanying resorption of the primary tooth root is sufficient to bring about the shedding of the tooth.

Occasionally, the relative position of the primary tooth and its permanent successor are such that the primary tooth root is not subject to conditions that induce resorption. In such cases, the permanent tooth may emerge into the oral cavity lingual to the primary tooth that it is supposed to replace. This condition is seen most often in the region of the mandibular incisors.

When the permanent tooth bud fails to develop, the roots of the primary tooth may resorb, even in the absence of a developing permanent successor, or the primary tooth may retain its roots and continue to function in the mouth for many years.

SUGGESTED READING

Gorski JP, Marks SC Jr. Current concepts of the biology of tooth eruption. Crit Rev Oral Biol Med 1992;3:185–206.

Kardos TB. The mechanism of tooth eruption. Brit Dent J 1996;181:91–94.

Marks SC. The basic and applied biology of tooth eruption. Connect Tissue Res 1995;32:149–157.

Marks SC Jr, Cahill DR. Experimental study in the dog of the non-active role of the tooth in the eruptive process. Arch Oral Biol 1984;29:311–322.

Steedle JR, Proffit WR. The pattern and control of eruptive tooth movements. Am J Orthod 1985;87:56–66.

14   *Temporomandibular Joint*

Only with a thorough knowledge of anatomy and occlusion can one begin to understand the functional movements of the mandible. Although the complex physiology and anatomy of the mandibular articulation and its associated muscles and ligaments are not reviewed in this text, some understanding of its design is necessary to appreciate the unique histologic composition of its parts.

ANATOMY

The *temporomandibular joint* is the articulation between the cranium and mandible (Figs. 14-1 and 14-2). The right and left joints of this bilateral articulation work as a unit; *within some limit of range,* its great adaptability permits virtually unrestricted movement of the mandible during speech and mastication. Proper functioning of the temporomandibular joint, with its effect on the occlusal contacts of the teeth, concerns nearly all phases of dentistry.

On either side of the head, the temporomandibular joint is made of two articulating bones—the *temporal bone* and the *mandible*—with an intervening *fibrous disc* and an enveloping *fibrous capsule*.

On the mandible, the articulating area is the upper anterior slope of the *mandibular condyle*. On the temporal bone of the cranium, the articulating areas are the *articular eminence* and the *anterior part of the mandibular fossa* (the *articular fossa*) (Figs. 14-2 and 14-3).

The mandibular fossa is a depression on the inferior aspect of the temporal bone, posterior and medial to the posterior end of the zygomatic arch. The tip of one's thumb fits into this space (Fig. 14-3). It is slightly broader mediolaterally than anteroposteriorly, and it is divided into anterior and posterior portions by the *petrotympanic fissure*. This fissure extends approximately from right to left near the posterior part of the fossa. The posterior part of the fossa, which is behind the fissure, is not involved in this joint. The anterior part of the mandibular fossa, which is anterior to the fissure, is also called the articular fossa. The anterior border of the articular fossa is a smooth, round ridge called the articular eminence, which is oriented mediolaterally and flattens anteriorly. The articular fossa and articular eminence are the parts of the temporal bone that comprise the cranial articulation of the temporomandibular joint. Locate these areas on Figure 14-3.

The condyle of the mandible (Fig. 14-4) fits into the articular fossa of the temporal bone when the jaws are closed (Figs. 14-2 and 14-3). Although during certain

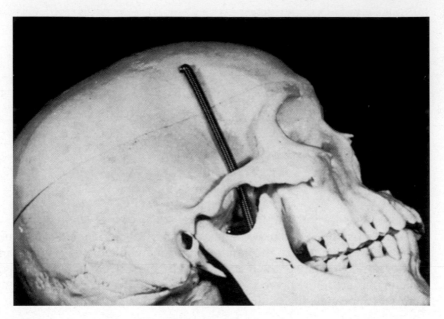

Figure 14–1. The right side of a human skull. Locate the mandible, condyloid process, zygomatic arch, and external auditory meatus, and notice their relation to the rest of the skull.

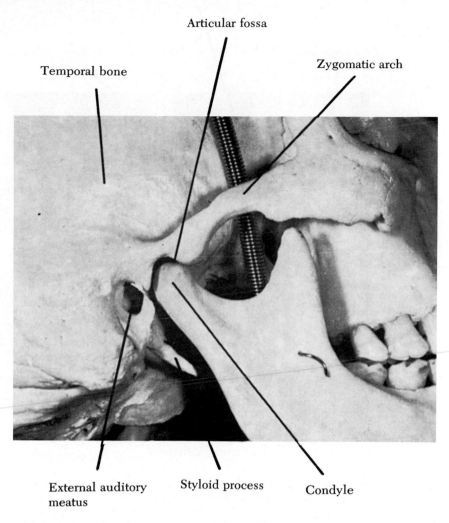

Articular fossa

Temporal bone

Zygomatic arch

External auditory meatus

Styloid process

Condyle

Figure 14–2. A closer view of the temporomandibular joint of the skull pictured in Fig. 14-1. If a human skull is available for study, compare it with these illustrations.

Articular eminence

Zygomatic arch

Articular fossa

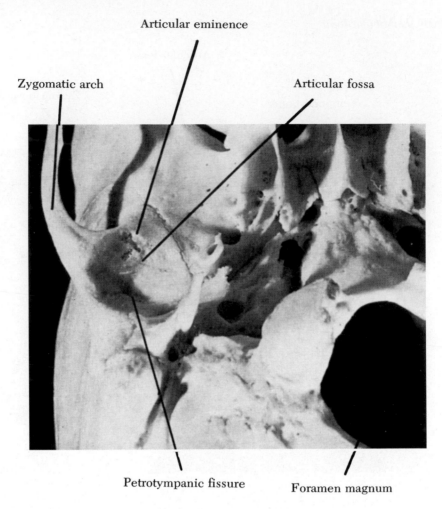

Petrotympanic fissure

Foramen magnum

Figure 14–3. Portion of the right side of the inferior surface of the skull pictured in Figs. 14-1 and 14-2. The right zygomatic arch (upper left) extends anteriorly (toward the top). Medial to its posterior end is a thumb-sized depression, the mandibular fossa. The anterior part of this fossa is called the articular fossa and is the area involved in the temporomandibular articulation.

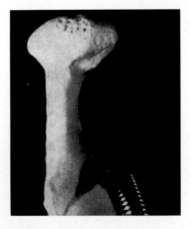

Figure 14–4. The superior anterior surface of the mandibular condyle. Notice how this condylar head will fit into the anterior part of the mandibular fossa (the articular fossa).

types of mandibular movements the condyle slides forward on the articular eminence, the surfaces of the condyle and eminence do not touch. Between them is the articular disc, which completely divides the temporomandibular joint cavity into upper and lower compartments (Fig. 14-5).

Figure 14-5 is a simplified diagram of the inside of this joint from the lateral aspect and represents the position of the joint components when the jaws are closed.

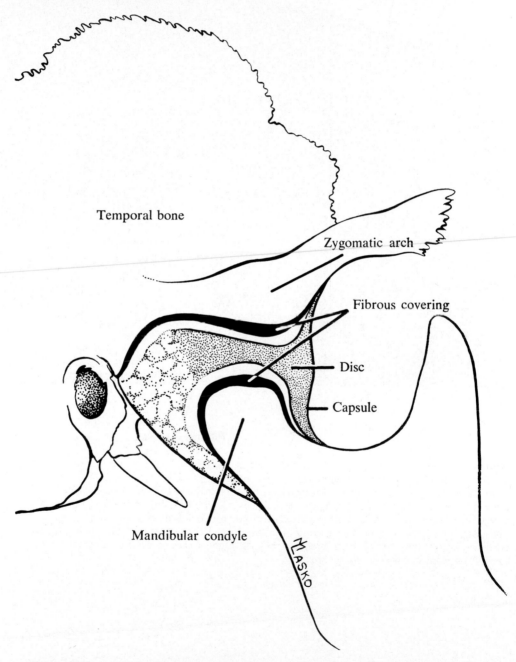

Figure 14–5. Diagram of the temporomandibular joint. Anterior is to the right of the picture. Compare this diagram with the photograph of the section of this joint in Fig. 14-7.

Upper space   Disc

Articular eminence

Temporal bone   Lower space   Articular fossa

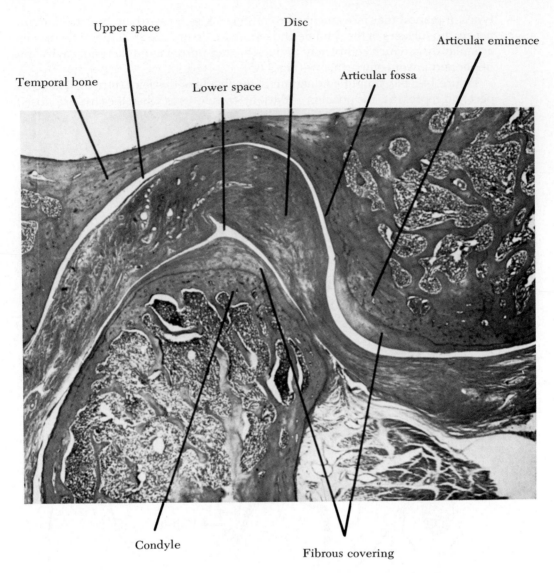

Condyle

Fibrous covering

Figure 14–6. Photomicrograph of a human temporomandibular joint. The specimen was removed in a block of tissue, fixed in formalin, demineralized, embedded in celloidin, sectioned at a thickness of about 25 microns, and stained with hematoxylin and eosin. This joint is seen from the lateral aspect. Anterior is toward the right of the picture; the white area across the top is the space of the brain case above the articular fossa. The condyle has a surface of compact bone, inside of which is the marrow cavity with bone trabeculae and bone marrow. The same kind of bone structure is seen in the articular eminence (upper right). Notice the difference in thickness of the fibrous covering on different parts of the articular fossa and mandibular condyle.

Compare this diagram with the picture of the skull in Figure 14-2; the *styloid process* is a good reference point for orientation. In the dry skull, there is no disc, and the condyle is in contact with the temporal bone. In live bone, as indicated by the diagram, the interposition of the articular disc forms an upper space (between disc and temporal bone) and a lower space (between disc and condyle). Notice that the mandibular condyle does not fit into the deepest part of the fossa; it remains somewhat forward, close to the eminence (Fig. 14-5). The disc is thin at its center, near the superior anterior surface of the condyle, and thicker at its edges. The capsule is seen here to enclose the joint anteriorly and posteriorly. Anteriorly, the disc and capsule are fused; posteriorly, the disc and capsule are connected by a pad of loose connective tissue that permits freedom of anterior movement. In this figure, the capsule encloses the joint somewhat like a stocking attached around the margin of the articular fossa and eminence (above) and around the circumference of the mandibular condyle (below).

The disc is attached to the lateral and medial sides of the mandibular condyle (Fig. 14-6) but is not attached to the temporal bone. When the mandible moves forward and back during functional movement, the disc, which is attached to the condyle, moves forward and back over the anterior surface of the articular fossa and eminence (Fig. 14-5). This gliding motion occurs in the upper compartment of the joint, between the disc and temporal bone. In the lower compartment of the joint, a different motion occurs in the form of a backward and forward swinging motion of the mandibular condyle against the underside of the disc. The attachment of the disc to the lateral and medial sides of the condyle is loose enough to permit this hinge-like movement of the mandible in the lower compartment of the joint.

If you place your fingertips on either side of your face, just in front of the tragus of the ear, you can feel some of the movements in this joint. First, open and close your mouth slightly several times, and notice the slight hinge-like movement in the joint. Second, open your mouth wide and close it; notice the forward movement of the condyle (with the disc attached, of course). Finally, place the tips of your little fingers in your ears, and move the mandible from side to side. The coordinated movements of the right and left joints are complex and are not described here. The interested student is referred to the extensive literature on this subject.

HISTOLOGY

The *capsule* of the temporomandibular joint is composed of two layers. The outer layer is relatively firm, fibrous tissue reinforced by the ligaments associated with the joint. The temporomandibular ligament on the lateral wall is particularly effective in controlling the extent of movement of the condyle.

The inner layer of the capsule, the *synovial membrane*, is a thin, connective tissue and contains blood vessels and nerves. *Synovial fluid* produced by this layer both lubricates the joint and furnishes nourishment to joint parts that are without a blood supply—the fibrous covering of the articulating surfaces of the bones and the center of the disc.

The *disc* is composed of fibrous connective tissue (Fig. 14-7). In older persons, the disc may contain a few chondrocytes (cartilage cells) and is referred to as *fibrocartilage*. Its shape is thin in the center and thick at the anterior and posterior borders. The center has no blood supply.

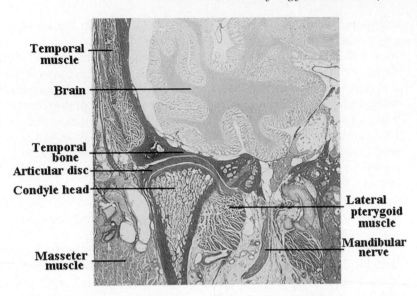

Figure 14–7. (See Color Plates) Frontal section through the human temporomandibular joint. Note the thinness of the temporal bone that separates the joint components from the temporal lobe of the brain.

On the temporal bone, the part enclosed by the capsule of the temporo-mandibular joint (i.e., the area of the articular fossa and eminence) is covered with fibrous connective tissue (Fig. 14-7). Notice that this fibrous layer is thicker at the posterior border of the eminence than in the articular fossa. Neither blood vessels nor nerves are found in this covering. Figure 14-8 is a frontal section of an adult temporomandibular joint through the level of the glenoid fossa. It shows some of the structures seen in the lateral view of Figure 14-7. Of special interest is the close relationship of the mandibular condyle to the temporal lobe of the brain.

On the mandibular condyle, the articulating surface is covered with fibrous con-nective tissue similar to that covering the temporal bone area (Fig. 14-7). A few chon-drocytes may be found in this layer, but there are no blood vessels or nerves. Notice that the fibrous layer is thick on the uppermost part of the curvature of the condyle.

The fibrous connective tissue that covers the bone surfaces of the temporo-mandibular joint makes this joint different from other, similar articulations. Most such movable joints contain a surface of hyaline cartilage rather than a layer of fi-brous connective tissue.

In the mandibular condyle of adults, compact bone is found beneath the fi-brous covering layer, and beneath this layer are the bone marrow and trabeculae (Fig. 14-7).

Figures 14-6 and 14-9 are photomicrographs of human fetuses at approximately 4 months in utero. Figure 14-6 was cut sagittally to reveal the lateral aspect of the joint. Figure 14-9 was cut in a direction perpendicular to the joint pictured in Fig-ure 14-6; in this section, the joint is seen from the front rather than from the side.

When compared with the adult temporomandibular joint, the fetal joint con-tains different histologic features. The articulating surfaces of the fetal joint are composed of dense, cellular connective tissue, and the articular disc is also highly cellular (Fig. 14-10).

Temporal bone   Upper space

Disc   Surface of
articular fossa

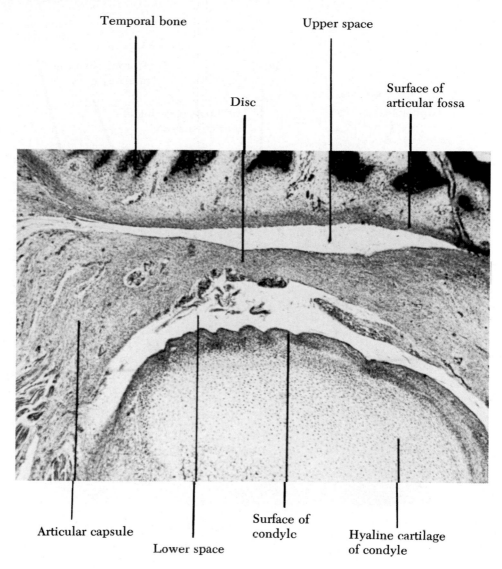

Articular capsule   Surface of
condyle
Lower space   Hyaline cartilage
of condyle

Figure 14–8. Lateral section of the temporomandibular joint of a human fetus at approximately 4 months in utero. Of interest is the soft cellular connective tissue of the articular disc. Compare this section with that of the adult temporomandibular joint seen in Fig. 14-7.

Hyaline cartilage
of condyle

Disc

Fibrous covering
of condyle

Fibrous covering of
articular fossa

Upper space

Lower space

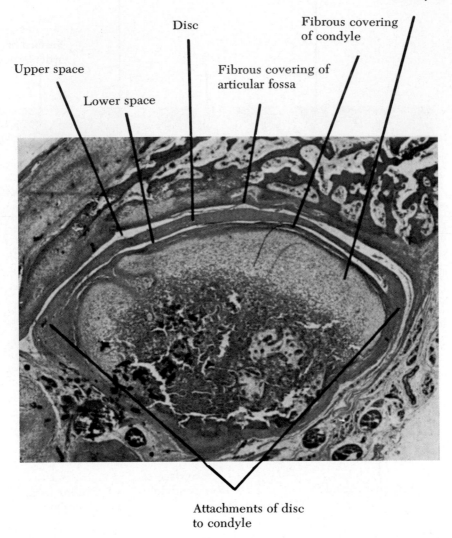

Attachments of disc
to condyle

Figure 14–9. Photomicrograph of a frontal section of the temporomandibular joint of a human fetus at approximately 4 months in utero. The disc is attached to the lateral and medial sides of the condyle. Because of the curvature of the bone, only the head of the condyle appears in this section. Notice the space above and below the disc and the fibrous covering of the surfaces of both the articular fossa and the condyle. Beneath the fibrous covering of the condyle of this fetus is cartilage. This area is one of the most long-lasting growth centers of the human body.

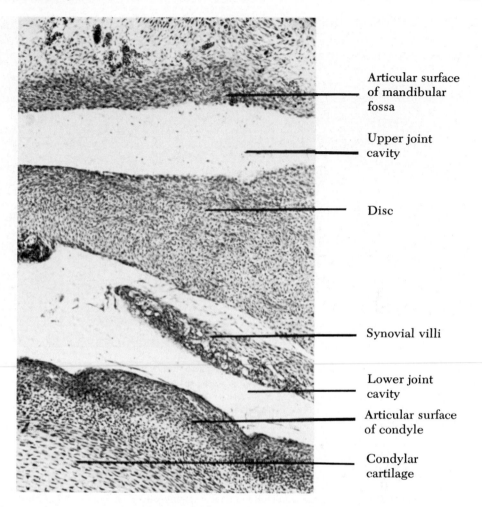

Articular surface
of mandibular
fossa

Upper joint
cavity

Disc

Synovial villi

Lower joint
cavity

Articular surface
of condyle

Condylar
cartilage

Figure 14–10. Higher magnification of the joint components seen in Fig. 14-6. Notice the dense cellular elements of the upper and lower articular surfaces and of the articular disc. Also note vascularity of the synovial villi seen in the lower space, which is a fold of the synovial membrane.

Beneath the cellular covering of the fetal condyle is hyaline cartilage (Figs. 14-9, 14-10, and 13-11). This is a growth center. At this location, the cartilage increases almost entirely by appositional growth (i.e., new cartilage added to existing cartilage edges) rather than by interstitial growth (i.e., cells within cartilage dividing) as in the ends of other bones (Fig. 14-11).

As development continues, the cartilage is gradually replaced by bone. Compact bone forms under the fibrous connective tissue covering, and trabecular bone replaces the cartilage within the mandibular head. The condyle takes on the adult histologic form, but this change does not happen early in life. The condylar cartilage persists and has growth potential until the individual is older than 20 years of age. It is the longest-lasting growth center of the body.

Growth of the condylar cartilage affects the height and length of the mandible and influences the shape of the entire face. To a large extent, the extent of growth in the mandibular condyle may determine the occlusion of the individual. Orthodontists refer to this type of occlusion as Class II and Class III occlusion.

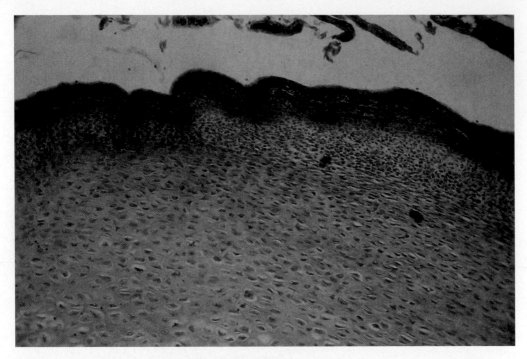

Figure 14–11. (See Color Plates) Higher magnification of the condylar process seen in Fig. 14-8. Cells of the dark-staining articular surface merge with cells of the underlying hyaline cartilage. Notice that the cells become larger as they pass from the articular surface to the cartilage; this characteristic is appositional growth. The space above the articular surface is the lower joint cavity. Compare with the adult joint in Figs. 14-6 and 14-7.

SELECTED READINGS

Sicher H, DuBrul EL. Sicher and DuBrul's Oral Anatomy. 8th ed. St. Louis (MO); Ishiyaku EuroAmerica; 1988.

LeResche L. Epidemiology of temporomandibular disorders: implications for the investigation of etiologic factors. Crit Rev Oral Biol Med 1997;8:291–305.

Sarnat BG, Laskin DM, eds. The Temporomandibular Joint: a biological basis for clinical practice. Philadelphia (PA): WB Saunders; 1992.

Index

Page numbers in *italics* denote figures; those followed by a t denote tables.